Atlas of Cutaneous Surgery

Atlas of Cutaneous Surgery

Neil A. Swanson, M.D.
Associate Professor of Dermatology and
Otolaryngology—Head and Neck Surgery,
Department of Dermatology,
University of Michigan Medical Center,
Ann Arbor, Michigan

Little, Brown and Company
Boston/Toronto

To Chris
For Bethany and Ingrid

Contents

Exercises

Preface

Welcome to cutaneous surgery. The first question you are probably asking is, "What is a dermatologist doing writing a book on cutaneous surgery?" This book is designed to be basic, and every physician—whether a surgeon or surgical subspecialist, dermatologist, family practitioner, internist, obstetrician-gynecologist, pediatrician, or emergency room physician— needs to know and has the opportunity to use basic surgical techniques and skills in his or her practice. This book is a self-instruction reference manual pertaining to basic surgical skills for physicians, physicians-in-training, and medical students.

Chapter 1, which deals with basic surgical techniques, began several years ago as an instruction manual for dermatology residents to teach them basic surgical skills using a pig's foot. Two years later, the advanced surgical techniques chapters were added as the skills of the residents increased and they demanded further instruction. In that form, it continued to be modified, clarified, and used to teach surgical techniques at the University of Michigan. In fact, during their required dermatology rotation, all third-year University of Michigan medical students are introduced to cutaneous surgery via a pig's foot session, like those described in this book.

Pigs' feet are the poor man's practice dummy. They are adequate for experimenting and practicing surgical techniques, but are in no way substitutes for real skin. They are useful for the entire book and can usually be purchased at a local meat market or grocery store. Two problems become apparent once one starts working on a pig's foot: There is a lack of elasticity to the tissue, and there is far less subcutaneous tissue than is contained in normal human skin. Nevertheless, pigs' feet are adequate for learning basic techniques and are readily available and relatively inexpensive. The fresher the pig's foot, the easier it is to use. As one moves on with more advanced techniques, other skin models may be better. The optimum would be obtaining access to fresh cadaver skin. There are also several foam and Elastoplast models that can be created on which to practice surgical techniques.

This book contains three chapters and five appendixes. Chapter 1, critical to the entire book, deals with the fundamentals of cutaneous surgery. These include instruments, excisions and incisions, the basic fusiform excision (the ellipse), the instrument tie, various undermining techniques, and methods of placing stitches from a simple interrupted stitch to more difficult running stitches. Chapter 1 finishes with basic variations on the fusiform excision and a series of practice tests. Within each subsection are exercises that will allow the student using this book to become facile with the techniques in question.

Chapter 2 deals with advanced surgical techniques, including local flaps. It begins with a discussion of the terminology and classification of basic, random pattern local flaps and then reviews the key basic techniques used whenever tissue movement occurs. Basic advancement, rotation, and transposition flaps are discussed in an exercise format. As in Chapter 1, a series of test exercises ends this chapter.

Chapter 3 also deals with advanced surgical techniques, namely, local skin grafts. This chapter introduces concepts of skin grafting and finishes with an exercise involving grafting techniques.

The appendixes contain important diagrams relating to relaxed skin tension lines, a discussion of local anesthesia and important anatomy related to anesthesia, available suture materials, and methods of hemostasis.

It is the goal of this book to help physicians discover the fun of cutaneous surgery, no matter what their status in the practice of medicine. With time, patience, and practice, the reader can enter the rewarding world of proper basic cutaneous surgery.

N. A. S.

Acknowledgments

Several acknowledgments are in order. These include my teachers, my students, and the personnel of the Mohs and Cutaneous Surgery and Oncology Unit at the University of Michigan.

Dr. William B. Taylor lit the flame that began my interest in cutaneous surgery while still a resident in dermatology at the University of Michigan. Drs. Samuel Stegman and Theodore Tromovitch kindled that flame and were very patient in conveying their knowledge to me during my fellowship at the University of California in San Francisco. The surgical subspecialty groups at the University of Michigan, who could have dampened the fire, have, in fact, kept it lit. My thanks to Drs. Charles Krause and Shan Baker of the Otolaryngology–Head and Neck Surgery Department, Drs. Reed Dingman and Louis Argenta of the Division of Plastic Surgery, and Dr. Bartley Frueh of the Ophthalmology Department.

I thank my students, in particular the residents in our department, who have been critical of me and my work and in review of the atlas as they used it. In particular, I would like to thank my fellows, Dr. John Stoner, Dr. Roy Grekin, Dr. Evelyn Vanderveen, and Dr. Christopher Zachary, for their critiques. Roy, now my associate, continues to do so on a daily basis.

Nancy Vargo, R.N., nurse clinician in the Mohs and Cutaneous Surgery and Oncology Unit, keeps me honest and critical of my own work. Cynthia Everling was very diligent in the preparation of the manuscript. Last but far from least, Mary Ann Olson of the Medical Illustration Department was very understanding and talented in her ability to interpret my words in her drawings and supplied the medical illustrations for this book.

Atlas of Cutaneous Surgery

1 Basic Techniques

Instruments

There are several instruments that are important in cutaneous surgery. They are all available from different companies in various sizes, shapes, and qualities. The student should become familiar with their uses and their names. Because quality varies, it is advisable for a surgeon on a tight budget to get a few instruments of good quality rather than several of poor quality. Good quality instruments will often last the lifetime of the surgeon.

SCALPELS

The scalpel has two parts, the knife handle and the blade. The two most common manufacturers are Bard Parker and Beaver. Bard Parker makes three commonly used blades: (1) No. 15, a convexly curved blade, used most commonly for excisional surgery; (2) No. 11, a sharp-pointed blade, used primarily for incision and drainage, and for some sharp dissection; and (3) No. 10, a blade shaped like the No. 15 but larger, used for large excisions and some shaves. These blades are illustrated in Figure 1. The differences in the sharpness of the No. 15 and No. 10 blades should be noted: the No. 15 blade is sharpest at the tip, whereas the No. 10 blade is sharpest at the belly.

Scalpels made by Beaver are smaller, extremely sharp, and are used for fine surgery. Their blades do not remain sharp for as long as the Bard Parker blades. Beaver scalpels are also illustrated in Figure 1, with several varieties and shapes shown.

Figure 1
Surgical instruments:
scalpels

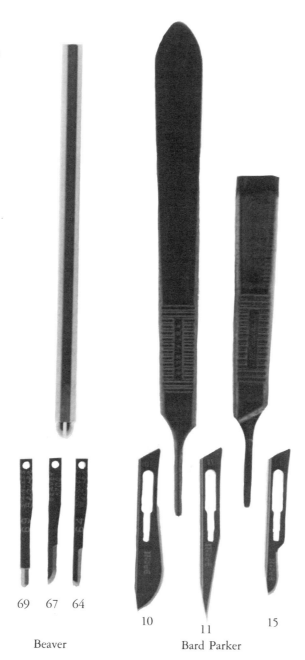

69 67 64

Beaver

10   11   15

Bard Parker

NEEDLE HOLDERS   Like scalpels, needle holders also come in a variety of sizes and shapes. The overall length of needle holders varies, as illustrated in Figure 2, and their tips also vary, from wide and blunt to very narrow and fine. Better quality needle holders have a diamond or hard-surfaced insert in their jaws. The jaws themselves can be either completely smooth or serrated. Some needle holders, as illustrated by the largest (A) in Figure 2, have scissors built into their handles or midportions, and are especially handy for surgery done when an assistant is not readily available. Needle holders with large jaws should be used with large needles; those with small jaws should be reserved for use with small-diameter needles. This is important, since large needles can damage or chip the inserts in small needle holders. The second needle holder (B) shown in Figure 2 is a small Webster needle holder, and the third (C) is the Castroveijo needle holder. I am particularly fond of the latter type, as it is very easy to use to quickly and accurately place small stitches, especially on the head and neck.

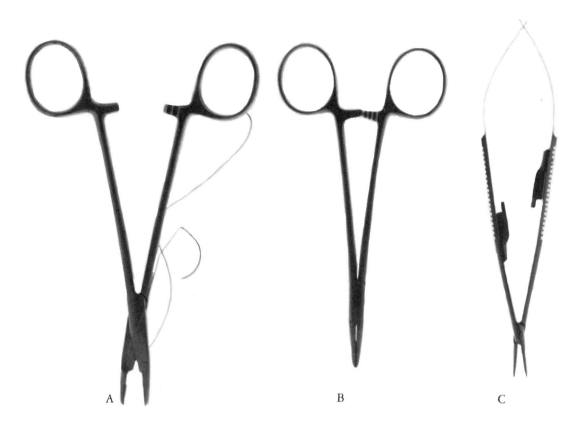

Figure 2
Surgical instruments:
needle holders

FORCEPS   Forceps, commonly called "pickups," are used for any type of surgery. They, too, come in various sizes and shapes. For cutaneous surgery, two basic types of forceps are required: one set should be toothed and the other should be smooth tipped. The toothed forceps I favor are the Addison or Brown Addison. Specialized forceps with curved tips or much finer forceps for plastic surgery–type procedures (e.g., those performed around structures such as the eye) are also available. These are illustrated in Figure 3.

Figure 3
Surgical instruments:
forceps

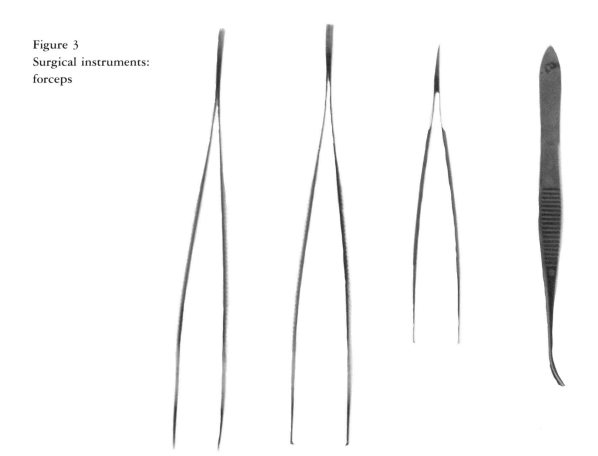

SCISSORS

Scissors also come in many sizes and shapes, and with many names. Perhaps the most common type are the Metzenbaum scissors, illustrated in Figure 4. These come in various lengths and are blunt tipped for use in cutting tissue and undermining. Good blunt-tipped undermining scissors are Castenares facelift scissors and another common type are Iris scissors, which are fine, sharp-pointed scissors with either curved or straight blades. They are used for fine work and dissection. Two other fine dissection scissors, with blunter tips, are Stevens Tonotomy scissors and Gradle scissors, both illustrated in Figure 4B. The Gradle scissors are my favorite for fine dissecting and undermining. The last scissors I should mention are suture and suture removal scissors (Figure 4D). These have a hooked end on one side that allows them to easily slip under a previously placed suture in order to remove it.

Figure 4
Surgical instruments:
scissors

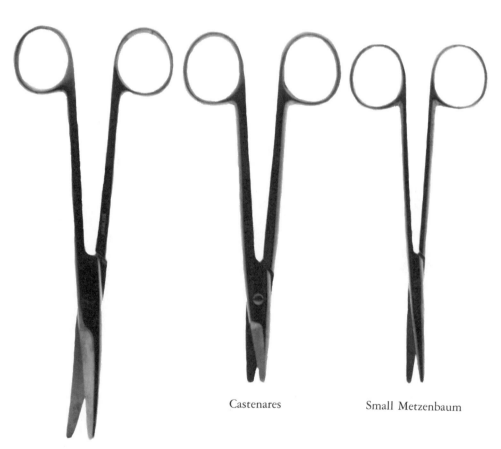

Castenares   Small Metzenbaum

Large Metzenbaum

A

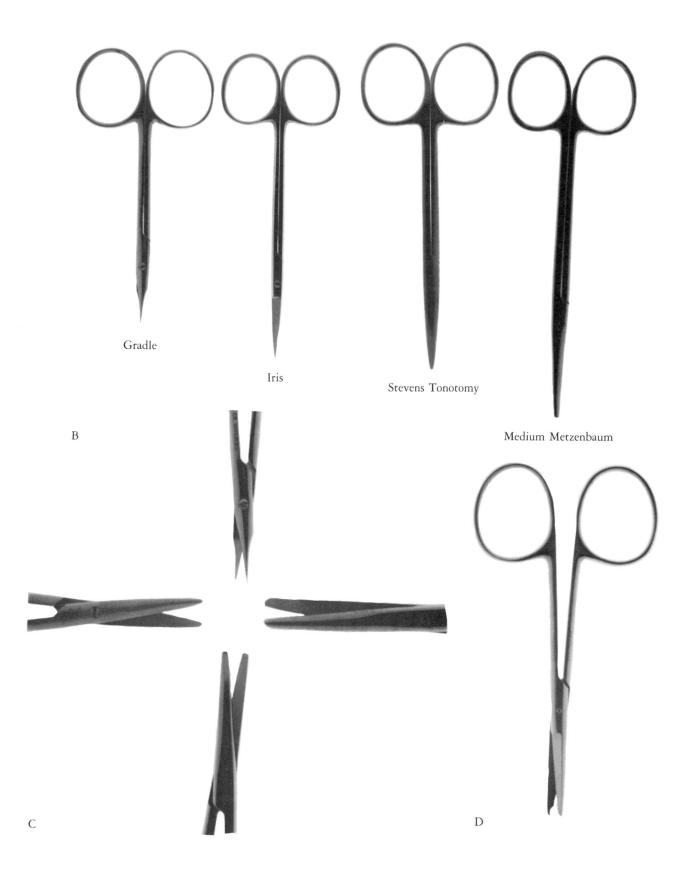

Gradle

Iris

Stevens Tonotomy

Medium Metzenbaum

B

C

D

SKIN HOOKS

Skin hooks are invaluable aides for atraumatic tissue handling and good cosmetic results. They are used to manipulate wound edges and retract skin. They vary in size, number of prongs at the tip, and sharpness of the prongs. The prongs vary in number, so that skin hooks range from single-pronged to three- and four-pronged "rake" hooks. These are illustrated in Figure 5.

PUNCHES

Punches come in different sizes and qualities for everyday use, and may be either disposable or reusable. Small punches, either power or hand driven, are available with diameters that begin at 1.5 mm and increase in 0.5-mm increments, to 6 mm. After 6 mm, punches increase in 1-mm increments to 10 mm. The smaller units are used for small punch replacements, punch elevations, and hair transplants. Punch biopsies generally require 3- or 4-mm disposable punches.

Figure 5
Surgical instruments
skin hooks

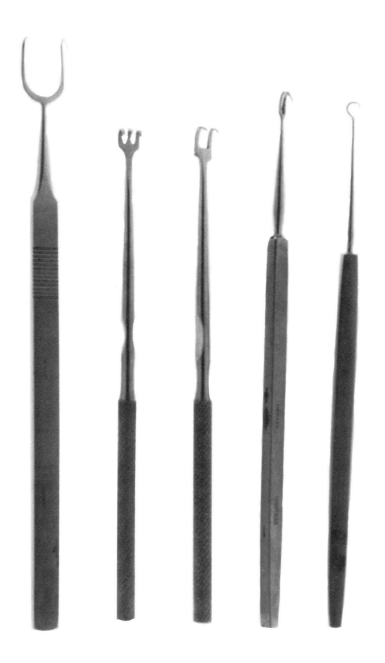

HEMOSTATS

Hemostats are also available in a range of sizes and shapes. The student should purchase one basic size with either a curved or straight tip. Hemostats are used primarily for clamping arterial bleeders or for blunt dissection, and should never be used to grasp skin edges needing suturing because they would traumatize wound edges and cause tissue damage.

SURGICAL PACK

For the exercises in this book, a typical surgical pack, as illustrated in Figure 6, is sufficient. It should include a Bard Parker handle with a No. 15 and a No. 10 blade, forceps with teeth, dissecting scissors such as the Metzenbaum scissors described earlier, suture scissors, a needle holder, and skin hooks. A marking pen or gentian violet is a valuable aid, as well. Sutures, which are discussed in detail in Appendix D, are available with large needles and in 3-0 and 4-0 sizes. When you have progressed to flaps, which are discussed in Chapter 2, you will find a caliper or ruler useful.

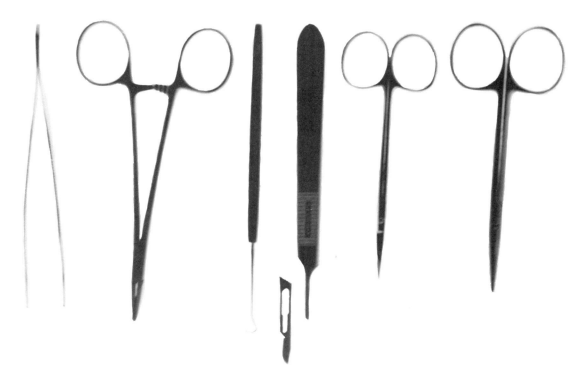

Figure 6
Surgical instruments:
surgical pack

Biopsies, Incisions, and Excisions

SHAVE BIOPSY OR EXCISION

The shave excision is an important skill for the practitioner. It is a fast, cosmetically acceptable, and practical means of removing a lesion or obtaining a biopsy. It is especially useful for raised or pedunculated lesions. There are two basic types of shaves: the superficial shave and the deeper roll shave. They differ only in depth, as their names imply. To begin a shave excision, inject local anesthesia into the area of the lesion. It is often useful to raise a "bleb" under the lesion that is similar to the bleb raised in a skin test (Figure 7B). This facilitates the shave. The lesion and surrounding tissue are then pinched up between the index finger and thumb, so that the lesion is raised, and the scalpel blade is passed under the lesion (Figures 7C and D). The depth of the shave is controlled by the angle of entry of the knife blade—the greater the angle, the deeper the shave. Bleeding is then controlled with either aluminum chloride solution or Monsel's solution (see Appendix E).

EXERCISE 1: THE SHAVE

1. Draw a lesion on the pig's foot.
2. Use a tuberculin syringe filled with saline solution to "anesthetize" the area, raising a bleb under the lesion.
3. Pinch the surrounding skin between thumb and index finger.
4. Perform a shave of the lesion by cutting underneath it at the appropriate angle, as illustrated in Figure 7.
5. Repeat until you are comfortable doing the procedure.

Figure 7
Shave biopsy or excision

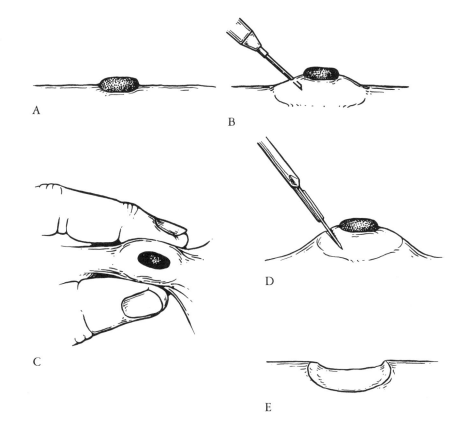

A

B

C

D

E

PUNCH BIOPSY OR EXCISION

The punch is a useful technique for the physician. It is a relatively safe, fast, and easy way to remove a piece of tissue for diagnosis or cosmesis. Cosmesis can be improved by making the circle of your punch into an oval by placing tension on the skin perpendicular to the desired long axis of the closure. After release, the elastic nature of the skin turns the circle into an oval, as illustrated in Figure 8. A trick in areas of neutral skin tension is to use a punch without placing tension on the skin. The circle remaining will then often align itself into an oval, showing the surgeon the direction of closure. My bias is that punch biopsies should be closed with suture.

EXERCISE 2: PUNCH BIOPSY OR EXCISION

1. Open a 3–4 mm punch and take note of its characteristics.
2. Place it on the pig's foot and, with your free hand, apply tension in a direction opposite to imagined skin lines.
3. Gently twist the punch into the skin to a desired depth, and remove.
4. **Gently** take hold of the plug of tissue with forceps, and cut beneath it at the deepest point with scissors.
5. Leave the hole to be closed in a later exercise.

Figure 8
Punch biopsy or excision

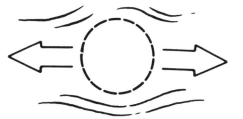 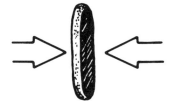

INCISION

Mastery of the incision is critical before moving on to any further excisional surgery. The incision should begin with the scalpel upright and perpendicular to the skin (Figure 9A). If any error is made, an external bevel of 10 degrees or less toward the lesion should be made (Figure 9B). As illustrated in Figure 9, one should generally avoid beveling the edges of an incision because this makes closure more difficult. There are a few special instances where beveling wound edges is valuable; however, for the vast majority of surgical incisions, beveling should be avoided. One example is illustrated in Figure 9C. When placing an incision in hair-bearing skin, beveling the incision across the hair follicles allows the hair to regrow through the scar, thus camouflaging it and preventing an area of alopecia. Using a rocking motion with countertension placed to firm the skin, a cut is made along the line of incision, as illustrated in Figure 10. Remember to use the sharp portion of the scalpel blades when making this cut. The exercise for incisions is incorporated into Exercise 3: Fusiform Excision (Ellipse).

Figure 9
Angle of incision

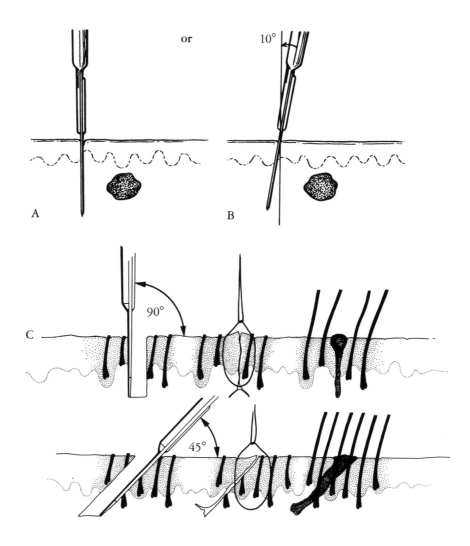

Figure 10
Rocking motion

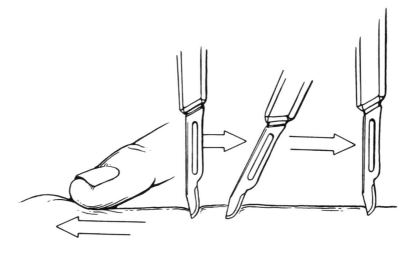

FUSIFORM EXCISION (ELLIPSE)

Fusiform excision or biopsy is the cornerstone of cutaneous surgery. It is easy to accomplish properly, gives excellent cosmetic results, obtains enough tissue of sufficient depth to give the pathologist the best chance for diagnosis, and can be accomplished quickly. The elliptical excision should always be diagrammed with its long axis corresponding to the relaxed skin tension lines (see Appendix B). The margins around a lesion will depend on whether the lesion is benign or malignant, being smaller when the lesion is benign. As a general rule, the length of an ellipse should be 3.0 to 3.5 times its width. This length-to-width ratio will vary, depending on anatomic location and elasticity of the skin. For example, on the elastic cheeks of an elderly patient, the length-to-width ratio can be small. On the same patient, over the nonelastic pretibeal surfaces of the lower legs, the length-to-width ratio may have to be as large as 5 : 1. Regardless of the length-to-width ratio, the ideal angle at the tip of an elliptical excision is 30 degrees. It has been shown that 30 degrees is the optimal angle at which to close without leaving a dog-ear, or pucker of redundant skin. As illustrated in Figures 11 and 12, several basic techniques are important to good cutaneous surgery. In summary, these are:

1. Diagram the lines of excision and follow them.
2. Keep the scalpel perpendicular to the skin (see Figure 9).
3. Use proper skin traction while cutting, and use a rocking motion, as shown in Figure 10.
4. Establish and stay in a uniform plane throughout the length of the excision.
5. Incise to the desired depth of excision **before** removing tissue. Remove tissue at a uniform depth, especially from the tips or apices of the ellipse.
6. Remove the ellipse, avoiding under-nicks (Figure 12). The ellipse can be removed with either sharp or blunt dissection. I prefer blunt dissection using scissors to better control the depth of tissue removal and to avoid nicking.

There are some tricks that may be used while performing the fusiform excision. If the beginner has difficulty making exact apices to the ellipse without nicking tissue, a No. 11 blade can be used to begin the ellipse. All of the fat at the tip of the ellipse should be removed. A common mistake is to remove a deeper portion of fat at the center of the ellipse, leaving fat in the apices of the ellipse. This creates a pseudo dog-ear, no matter how well designed the ellipse is. Blunt removal of tissue often allows for undermining, which will be discussed later in this chapter, at the same time the ellipse is removed.

**EXERCISE 3:
FUSIFORM EXCISION
(ELLIPSE)**

1. Make two or three straight incisions, using a rocking motion with a scalpel as shown in Figure 10. Leave these for a future exercise. Draw a 3–5 mm × 3–5 mm hypothetical lesion with a marking pen or gentian violet.

2. Diagram incision lines so as to keep a 3 : 1 ratio of length to width, with the ideal 30-degree angle at the apices. On the pig's foot, as on the extremities of a patient, it is better to err in making the ellipse too long or too narrow than too short or too wide, because of the lack of tissue movability in the skin of human extremities or in pig's skin.

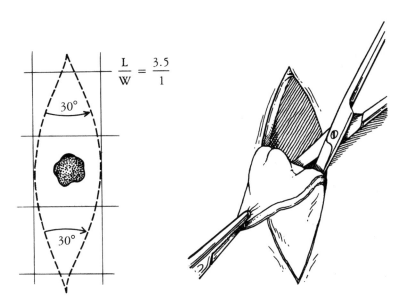

Figure 11
Ellipse

Figure 12
Removing the ellipse

Closure of the ellipse is more difficult if the ellipse is too short or wide.

3. Using a No. 15 blade, cut both sides of the ellipse to an equal depth, keeping the knife handle perpendicular to the skin or tipped 10 degrees toward the lesion. Remember to use the sharpest part of the Bard Parker blade when performing the incision.

4. Begin at whichever end of the ellipse is more comfortable for you, and gently dissect in one plane to remove the tissue. Perform this action with sharp dissection and try it again elsewhere on the pig's foot with blunt dissection to see which you prefer.

5. Repeat at least twice, varying the width and length of your ellipse.

6. Leave these incisions for future exercises.

Instrument Tie

The square knot is the basic surgical knot and should be used in **all** cutaneous surgery. Decent results may be obtained with the granny knot occasionally, but not reliably. The square knot is easy to perform and can be done quickly, but should always be done carefully.

**EXERCISE 4:
INSTRUMENT TIE
SQUARE KNOT**

1. Using the practice incisions left from Exercise 3, place a suture in any way desired, leaving about 4–5 cm (1.5–2.0 in.) on the short end of the suture.

2. Take up slack, with the needle end (long end) of the suture in the palm of your hand.

3. Bringing the needle holder across the wound from the short end to the long end of the suture, loop the suture twice around the tip of the needle holder (Figure 13A).

4. Open the needle holder, grasp the short end of the suture, and gently pull the loops off the needle holder and reverse your hands (Figures 13B and C).

5. **Stop!** Look carefully to see which way the double loop will lay most evenly and pull most snugly. This knot should be slightly looser than the ultimate tension desired on the wound, as the second knot will slightly tighten the tie.

6. If necessary, reverse the short and long ends of the suture to lock the first stitch.

7. Bring the needle holder across the wound from the short end into the long end of the suture, make a single loop (Figure 13D), and again grasp the short end (Figure 13E), pull the loop off the needle holder, and reverse your hands (Figure 13F).

Figure 13
Instrument tie and
square knot

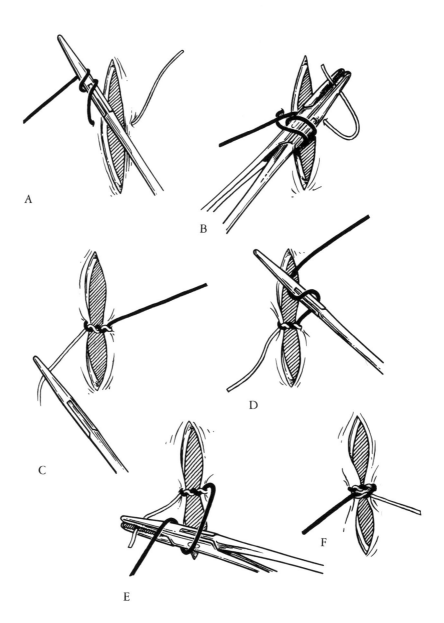

A

B

C

D

E

F

8. **Stop!** Again, carefully look to make sure your knot is even and square to the first knot before tightening—then tighten.
9. Repeat steps 7 and 8.
10. Practice this technique several times on the incisions made in Exercise 3.

Undermining

Undermining is important both to relieve tension on a wound and to free wound edges for eversion. It can be done in any tissue plane, depending on the location of the wound; undermining is usually more superficial on the face and deeper on the trunk, for example. On the pig's foot there is little subcutaneous tissue, but the principles of undermining nevertheless can be learned.

Undermining can be accomplished using either sharp dissection with a surgical blade or blunt dissection with scissors. If a tissue plane on the face can be readily identified, blunt undermining with scissors can prevent unwanted nicks or exiting from the plane that can occur in sharp undermining with a surgical blade.

There is no hard and fast rule for the amount a surgeon should undermine, but a general rule of thumb is to undermine each side one-half the length of the incision. If tension persists on wound edges, undermine further before revising your excision. Skin hooks should always be used so that wound edges are handled atraumatically (Figure 14).

EXERCISE 5:
UNDERMINING

1. Use the deepest of your practice elliptical excisions from Exercise 3.
2. Identify a plane and undermine 1 cm back, using the scalpel on one side and scissors on the other. Use your skin hook to handle wound edges.
3. The skin hook should be held like a pencil, placing the third or fourth finger on the skin to identify the depth to be undermined and to provide pressure on the surface against which to undermine.
4. Repeat with a second excision.

Figure 14
Undermining

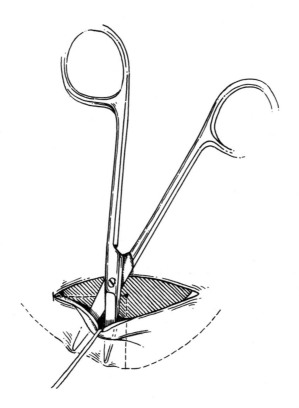

Simple Interrupted Stitch

The simple interrupted stitch is the most fundamental and common stitch used in cutaneous surgery. It can anchor a wide wound well, finely evert the edges of a narrow wound, and precisely close a wound with edges of unequal height. When this stitch is properly performed, the flask shape of the needle and suture path will gently and evenly evert the edges of the wound (Figures 15B and C). (When the stitch is performed incorrectly, the wound edges are inverted rather than everted, as demonstrated in Figure 15A.) Wounds with one edge higher than the other can be closed by varying the depth of the suture (shallow on high side, deeper on low side as in Figure 15F). The length of the wound that is closed by one stitch will vary according to the size of the bite, or distance from the needle pass to the incision (Figure 15D). The larger the bite, the greater the wound length closed with one stitch.

Disadvantages of the simple interrupted stitch include: (1) "railroad-track" scarring, (2) occasional inversion of the wound edges, and (3) the fact that it is time consuming. The first two of these disadvantages can be minimized by careful placement of sutures—making sure wound edges are everted and equal on each side. The proper tension is important, as too tight a stitch causes puckering and can accentuate railroad tracks. Proper timing of suture removal is also important. A good rule of thumb is to gently "kiss" the everted wound edges.

EXERCISE 6: SIMPLE INTERRUPTED STITCH

1. Using the first ellipse made in Exercise 3, begin closing with the simple interrupted stitch.
2. For most wounds, beginning to stitch in the middle of the wound and following the rule of halves (see Figure 31B) provides good, even closure.
3. Place the needle in the needle holder and begin your stitch with the needle tip perpendicular to the skin. The needle should be held in the tip of the needle holder, one-third of the way down the needle curve. This gives the best control without bending the needle.
4. Go through both sides of the wound in one motion if possible, exiting the skin directly opposite and at the same distance from the wound margin as the entrance (Figure 15D).
5. If necessary, this stitch can be done in two motions, as shown in Figure 15C.
6. By using your finger or forceps, you can help the needle exit less traumatically.

Figure 15
Simple interrupted stitch

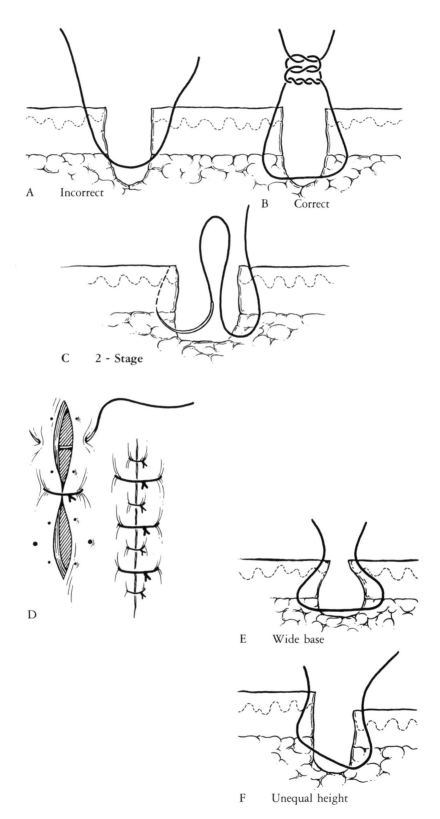

A   Incorrect

B   Correct

C   2 - Stage

D

E   Wide base

F   Unequal height

7. Tie an instrument square knot, as described in Exercise 4.

8. If properly done, the flask-shaped path of the suture and proper tension on the knot should result in a nicely everted wound edge.

9. Repeat the procedure until the excision is closed, varying the size of the bite (distance from the suture line). Remember that a wider bite closes a larger length of the wound and a smaller bite, a smaller length.

Suture Removal

Suture-removal technique is often unappreciated, but is as important as careful wound closure. Improper suture removal can undo even the most careful closure by placing tension on the suture line in a way that can reopen skin edges and cause dehiscence of the wound. The correct method of suture removal is illustrated in Figure 16. The surgeon should cut the suture and then pull the freed knot across the suture line (Figure 16A). This pulls the suture out in the direction in which it was placed, and avoids putting unwanted tension opposite the axis of the closed wound edge. If the suture is pulled out away from the closure line, wound dehiscence may result (Figure 16B).

EXERCISE 7: SUTURE REMOVAL

1. Remove the interrupted stitches placed in Exercise 6 by cutting the suture and then pulling the knot and suture across the axis of the closed wound.

2. When removing sutures in the remaining exercises, **always** use this technique. Be sure to practice it correctly.

Figure 16
Suture removal

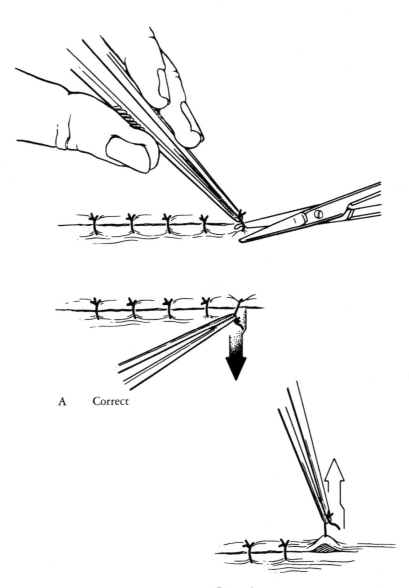

A   Correct

B   Incorrect

Vertical Mattress Stitch

CLASSIC

The vertical mattress stitch can be used in many circumstances. Properly placed, it everts skin edges better than any other stitch. It can also be used to close dead space in a wound with or without the need for subcutaneous stitches. It is a strong stitch that can provide added support to a lesion under stress or provide a "stay" suture to initially approximate and align a wound to be closed using other types of stitches. Surgeons debate the use of this stitch on the face; its opponents feel that face wounds should always be approximated with subcutaneous sutures first for best cosmetic results. I feel that the vertical mattress stitch is invaluable on any part of the body, since when properly done it approximates everted edges with less tension than any other stitch. It might be performed on the face in areas where wound edges naturally tend to invert, such as in a forehead skin crease.

Disadvantages of the vertical mattress stitch are few. The main one is that stitch placement is time consuming, especially when care is taken to perform it properly; it can cause "railroad tracking" if done with insufficient care.

Some notes on the mechanics of the stitch are in order (Figure 17): (1) the deep stitch goes in first; (2) this first "bite" should be of equal distance from the respective wound edges (that distance varies depending on tension on the wound and the amount of dead space to be closed); (3) the second, shorter bite should also be of equal distance from the wound edges to provide even eversion; (4) the edges of the wound should be gently and evenly pulled together to provide equal tissue approximation at all levels of the incision; (5) equal tension should be placed on each stitch; and (6) if necessary, the deep bite can pick up the deepest portion of the wound, which helps to close all dead space.

EXERCISE 8: VERTICAL MATTRESS STITCH

1. Use the second excision site from Exercise 3. The amount of tension on the wound will determine the distance from the edges your first (deep) stitch must go (the greater the tension, the deeper the bite).
2. Plan your suturing—begin in the middle of the wound and use the rule of halves.
3. Again with the needle perpendicular to the skin, make the first deep bite on both sides of the wound equidistant from the wound edges, as shown in Figure 17. If necessary, come out in the middle of the

Figure 17
Vertical mattress stitch

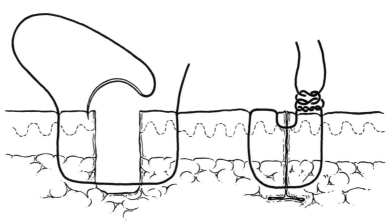

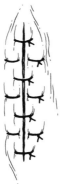

Vertical mattress alternating with interrupted stitches

wound and regrasp the needle to finish the stitch, as shown in Figure 15C.

4. Grasp the needle in the middle, to shorten the curve, and place a shallow interrupted stitch approximately 1 mm from each edge in the opposite direction of the first pass.

5. Tie your first knot (see Figure 13) and gently tighten the suture with slow, even pressure. Lock it if necessary.

6. Place your next two knots squarely.

7. Repeat the procedure until the wound is closed.

VARIATIONS

The **half-buried vertical mattress stitch** does not provide as much tension as the vertical mattress stitch, but can be used to close dead space and may be stronger than the simple interrupted stitch, with a better cosmetic result. As you can see in Figures 18A and C, one side of the stitch is subcuticular so that no needle marks are left on that side of the wound when healed. Thus, this stitch is of special value on the face near hair-bearing skin, where one side of the scar will be hidden (e.g., by eyebrows or sideburns) and the other will not. It is also of value on tips of flaps as a tip stitch (see Figure 19).

The **near-far adaptation of the verticle mattress stitch** has the advantage of elevating the deep tissue in which it is placed. An example of a good use for this stitch is suturing the obicularis muscle in a lip wedge (see Figure 39). The stitch is placed by beginning as in the classic vertical mattress stitch (see Figure 17), but exiting at the epicuticular site (Figure 18B). Then, reversing the direction of the needle, begin another deep bite in the same side just exited. Exit again on the other side of the wound with another small epicuticular bite.

The **three-point corner (tip) stitch** is an important variation of the vertical mattress stitch. As shown in Figure 19, improper placement of this stitch can result in tip necrosis (Figure 19A). The stitch can be placed in two ways. The first is shown in Figures 19B and C, passing subcuticularly through the "tip" to be closed. The second, shown in Figures 19D and E, is actually a very superficial interrupted stitch placed through the "tip."

EXERCISE 9: HALF-BURIED VERTICAL MATTRESS STITCH

1. Use the third excision from Exercise 3.

2. Begin your first (deep) bite as in the vertical mattress stitch but come out through the center (open area) of the wound and regrasp the needle with the needle holder about three-fourths of the way from the tip.

Figure 18
Variations of the vertical
mattress stitch

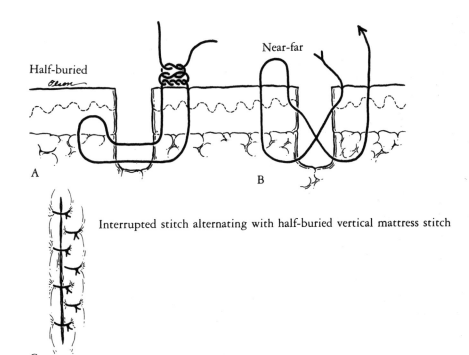

A Half-buried

B Near-far

Interrupted stitch alternating with half-buried vertical mattress stitch

C

3. Continue as you would in the vertical mattress stitch, but do not puncture the skin.

4. Instead, pull the needle tip back so that it exits subcuticularly (or intradermally) on the pig's foot.

5. Come through the initial (opposite) edge, tie your initial knot, and gently tighten it to evert the edges, as before.

6. Close the wound using this stitch, alternating every other or every third stitch with the regular vertical mattress stitch for comparison (Figure 18C).

EXERCISE 10: THREE-POINT CORNER (TIP) STITCH

1. Make a **V** incision in the pig's foot as diagrammed in Figure 19 and undermine.

2. Starting on the right-hand side of the incision, begin an interrupted stitch in the direction of the tip, but exit middermally in the tissue before completing the stitch (Figure 19B).

3. Pass the needle intradermally through the tip.

4. Pass the needle back through the left side of the incision, beginning middermally and exiting in skin across from original point of entrance.

5. Gently tie (Figure 19C).

6. You now have completed a **Y–V**-plasty. This stitch is critical and is used a great deal in Chapter 2.

7. A second option in this stitch is shown in Figures 19D and E. Recent work has shown that placement of this stitch as a superficial interrupted stitch allows the suture pass to actually parallel the dermal plexus of vessels, thereby causing less ischemia at the tip than the stitch illustrated in Figure 19A. Therefore, this stitch is acceptable as long as it is placed superficially.

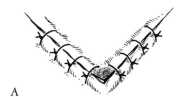

Figure 19
Three-point corner (tip) stitch

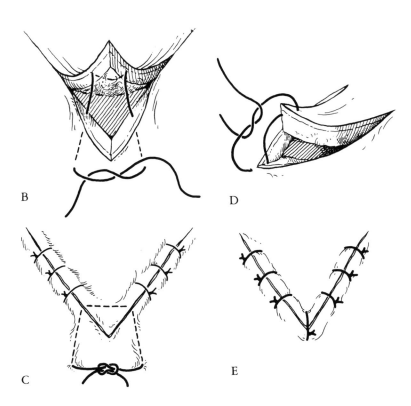

A

B   D

C   E

Horizontal Mattress Stitch

CLASSIC

The horizontal mattress stitch is invaluable as a "stay" stitch, when closing a wound or approximating wound edges for completion of the closure with a second, more superficial interrupted stitch. It is usually placed deeply and at a good distance from the wound edges. It also can provide hemostasis in a bleeding wound.

The interval of time for the removal of this stitch is variable. It may be removed at the time of surgery when suturing is complete, a few days later when wound healing has begun, or, if tension is sufficient, it may be left in place as a "stay" for a few weeks. If the latter is the case, it should be bolstered, as illustrated in Figure 20, to keep it from cutting into the skin. Another problem may arise if this stitch is pulled too tightly, which results in tissue hypoxia and thus poor healing.

Figure 20
Classic horizontal
mattress stitch

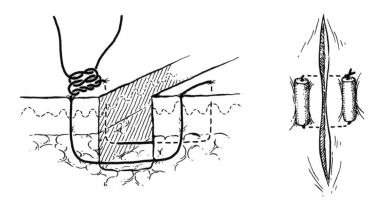

VARIATIONS

Illustrated in Figure 21, the **canal stitch** is a variation of the horizontal mattress stitch that actually inverts the wound edge where it is placed. It is used to close and evert the deep edge and/or the mucosal surface when suturing from the outside (cutaneous side) of a wound. By inverting the wound edge, the mucosal surface is everted. The basic technique for this stitch is illustrated in Figure 21, but it is really just the routine horizontal mattress stitch placed in the reverse direction.

The **half-buried horizontal mattress stitch (four-point corner [tip] stitch)** is used for T-type closures. It can also be used, like the half-buried vertical mattress stitch, to hide one side of the suture in a subcuticular plane without leaving exit marks in the skin. It is best illustrated in Figure 22.

EXERCISE 11: HORIZONTAL MATTRESS STITCH AND VARIATIONS

1. Make a careful elliptical excision (as in Exercise 3) that is at least 5 cm (2 in.) long.
2. Begin an interrupted stitch in the middle of the wound (Figure 20).
3. Move approximately 3 mm laterally, reverse the needle in the needle holder, and make a second bite equidistant from the wound edges, like the first stitch. Your second stitch should be parallel to your first and should be placed in the opposite direction.
4. Tie with gentle pressure—if tension on the wound is great, you may wish to use a fourth knot. If desired, use a small piece of cotton, or cardboard from a suture packet, as a bolster.
5. Next, place a canal stitch by reversing the direction of the pass of your needle, as shown in Figure 21. Make the first pass parallel to the axis of the wound, cross to the opposite side, reverse the needle in the needle holder, and make another pass parallel to the axis of the wound.
6. Tie the knot in the usual position, inverting the skin surface of the wound and everting the undersurface.

EXERCISE 12: FOUR-POINT CORNER (TIP) STITCH

1. Make a T incision in the pig's foot, as shown in Figure 22, and undermine.
2. Starting above the top of the T, begin an interrupted stitch to the right of the intersection, as in Figure 22A.
3. Exit the stitch in the middermis, regrasp the needle, and make a middermal stitch through the edges of the intersection of the T, as in Figures 21B and C.

Figure 21
Canal stitch

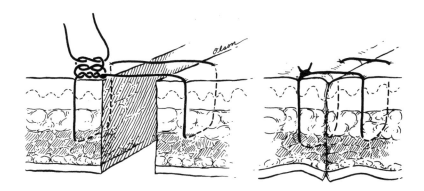

·**Figure 22**
Half-buried four-point
corner (tip) stitch

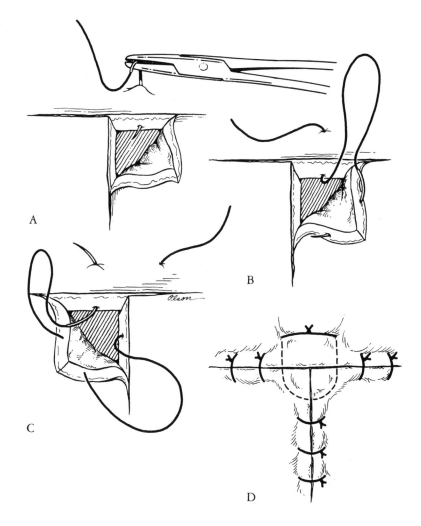

4. Finish with a deep stitch, entering in the middermis and exiting to the left of the entrance stitch, equidistant from the skin edge (Figure 22D).

5. Gently tie the knot. This stitch, along with the three-point corner (tip) stitch, will be used extensively in Chapter 2.

Subcutaneous Stitch (Buried Stitch)

The subcutaneous stitch is important for providing wound stability, closing dead space, and—if placed properly—helping to evert the edges and relieve tension on the wound.

It is important to remember several points of techniques when using this stitch: (1) do not pull the stitch too tightly or tissue necrosis can result; (2) most of the time a stitch placed only in fat will pull through when tied or stressed—therefore, try to include a portion of dermis or fascia with the stitch; (3) because the major purpose of this stitch is to close dead space, make sure your final product is deep enough. The subcutaneous stitch is **not** meant to be subcuticular and, if placed that high, will have a tendency to pucker wound edges or spit suture through the final wound.

Knot placement is important in this stitch. Instrument ties can be difficult, especially in deep wounds where traction near the knot is needed to approximate the tissue. Also, with plain-gut or chromic-gut suture, which is friable (especially when old), the needle holder applied to the suture will weaken and break it; this makes instrument ties even more difficult. Therefore, review hand-tying, as this can be the easiest and most secure way to tie these knots. When tying the knot, pull parallel to the axis of the wound to help get the best tissue approximation possible.

The position of the knot is also important (Figure 23). In very deep wounds, the knot can be positioned upward without undue tissue reaction (Figures 23A and C). However, in the wounds you will be making on the pigs' feet and when performing cutaneous surgery, the subcutaneous stitch will be more superficial and the knot should be buried (Figures 23B and D).

EXERCISE 13: SUBCUTANEOUS STITCH (BURIED STITCH)

1. Use an undermined excision, as explained in Exercise 5.

2. The position of the knot will depend on the direction of the first bite (see Figure 23). Figure 23A: Needle point down with first bite yields a knot up. Figure 23B: Needle point up with the first bite yields a knot down, or "buried."

Figure 23
Subcutaneous stitch
(buried-knot)

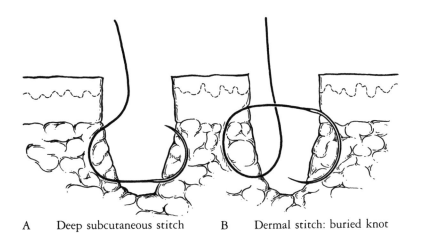

A   Deep subcutaneous stitch   B   Dermal stitch: buried knot

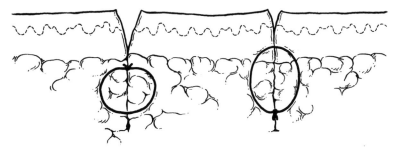

C   Upward knot placement,   D   Buried knot placement,
    acceptable for deep wounds   correct for dermal wounds

3. The mechanics of this stitch are the same as those of the simple interrupted stitch (see Exercise 6 and Figure 15).

4. Close the wound, alternating knots up and down and making sure your stitch is deep enough. Remember to pull parallel to the axis of the wound when tying the knots.

5. Practice both hand and instrument ties to see which is more satisfactory to you.

6. Close the wound practicing any stitch with which you feel **un**comfortable.

Running Stitches

Running stitches, whichever method is used, are a convenient, rapid means of suturing well-approximated tissue with equal wound edges on which little tension is placed. Running stitches are valuable on eyelids, neck, scrotum, or whereever loose skin is found. They should not be placed deeply, or where dead space has not previously been closed. It is important to place one end of the stitches perpendicular to the suture line. Running stitches can be used to apply equal tension rapidly to wound edges and to obtain final eversion of wound edges. The running horizontal mattress stitch is especially good for these purposes.

The running subcuticular stitch is the most difficult of the running stitches to master. However, when used properly, it provides superior cosmetic results because it leaves no suture exit and entrance marks along the edge of the suture line. The running subcuticular stitch should be used only on excisions where the wound is well approximated, the edges are everted, any dead space has been eliminated, and wound tension is minimal. This stitch can be left in place for long periods of time and should be placed using a monofilament suture such as Prolene (see Appendix D). There are several ways to anchor the loose ends of the stitch. One method is to pull the end of the suture to the desired tension, place the loose suture ends in Mastisol (or tincture of benzoine), and affix them with a Steri-strip. My favorite method is to tie the ends back on themselves.

For ease of suture removal, a long wound should have an exit point from the subcuticular stitch every 2 to 3 cm, as diagrammed in Figure 27. This is sometimes called leaving an extracutaneous loop of suture.

After placing a running subcuticular stitch, there are often a few small gaps left along the suture line. These may be sutured using very shallow, interrupted stitches, called epicuticular stitches, or by placing a second, more superficial, running subcuticular stitch. The following exercises explain these stitches in detail.

EXERCISE 14: BASIC RUNNING STITCH

1. Make a long (5 cm or 2 in.), narrow excision in the pig's foot.
2. Begin at whichever end you prefer and make an interrupted stitch. Tie with instrument (Figure 24).
3. Cut the **short** end only.
4. Make evenly placed interrupted passes with the needle for the length of the wound, keeping each pass perpendicular to the suture line.
5. With the last stitch, leave a loose "loop" to use in the tie.
6. Begin the tie as in Exercise 4, only grasp the loop (both strands) instead of a free end when laying down the knot.
7. Finish the knot.

Figure 24
Basic running stitches

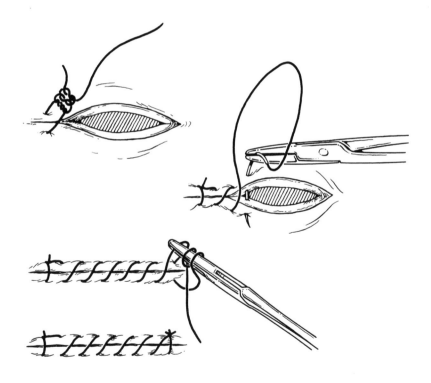

**EXERCISE 15:
RUNNING LOCKED
STITCH**

1. Make a new excision, or remove the sutures from an old one. Begin the stitch as in steps 2 and 3 in Exercise 14.

2. Put tension on the long end of the stitch with your odd hand, and pass the needle as if making the next stitch (Figure 25).

3. As the needle tip exits the skin, make a loop with your odd hand, pass the needle-holder tip through this loop, grasp the needle point, and pull through the loop creating a "locked" stitch.

4. Repeat steps 2 and 3 for the length of the wound.

5. Place your last stitch **without** the lock, as in Exercise 14, so as to leave a looped end with which to tie.

6. Tie as in Exercise 14.

Figure 25
Running locked stitch

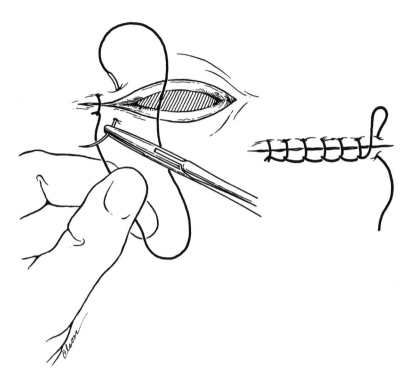

EXERCISE 16: RUNNING HORIZONTAL MATTRESS STITCH

1. Begin as in Step 1 in Exercise 15.

2. Beginning at one end of the excision, place an interrupted stitch. Cut both strands, but leave one longer than the other.

3. Now, begin at the opposite end of the wound, and place and tie an interrupted stitch. Again, leave one strand of the suture long.

4. Place an interrupted stitch, exiting on the opposite side of the wound (Figure 26).

5. Reverse the needle in the needle holder and, beginning on the same side from which you exited, place an interrupted stitch.

6. Again, reverse the needle in the needle holder and place an interrupted stitch in the opposite direction to which the last stitch was placed.

7. Continue this procedure for the length of the wound, until the opposite end is reached.

8. Using the suture end, which you left long in step 2, finish this stitch by tying it to the loose end of the suture. This is an excellent way to finish a running stitch, if you think far enough in advance to leave the loose end long when placing the interrupted stitch. It prevents the bulky knot that results when a running stitch is tied back onto a loop as in Exercises 13 and 14.

Figure 26
Running horizontal
mattress stitch

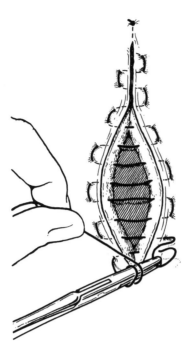

EXERCISE 17:
RUNNING
SUBCUTICULAR
STITCH

1. Remove suture and use the incision from Exercise 14 or 15.

2. Begin at one end of the wound, approximately 1 cm opposite the apex of the ellipse.

3. Make a bite, as if placing an interrupted stitch exactly at the apex of the excision.

4. Select one edge of the wound, and make a subcuticular bite parallel to the skin surface.

5. Make a similar bite, backspacing slightly, in the opposite edge of the wound.

6. Continue this procedure, exiting the skin (as shown in Figure 27) after you have gone 2 cm, until you reach the other apex of the excision. Remember to backspace slightly, as this is critical to fine, equal eversion of the wound edges.

7. Make your last bite, with the needle pointing upward, at the apex. Exit the skin approximately 1 cm opposite the apex.

8. Pull gently to approximate the wound.

9. Anchor the ends by tying the suture back on itself.

10. If there is a small gap in the closure line, approximate it using a fine epicuticular interrupted stitch.

Figure 27
Running subcuticular
stitch

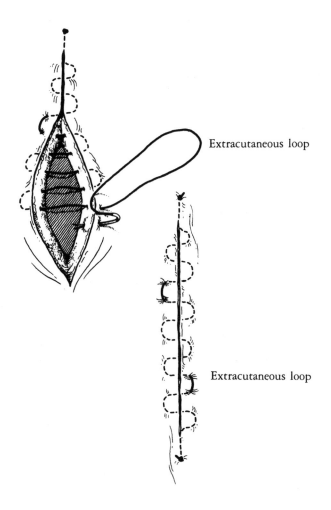

Extracutaneous loop

Extracutaneous loop

Dog-Ear Repair

No matter how careful the surgeon is, a pucker of redundant skin or "dog-ear" is often left at one or both wound ends. As this is particularly true in beginning flap surgery, the technique for dog-ear repair will be discussed again in Chapter 2. The dog-ear repair technique is critical to good cutaneous surgery.

Whatever method is used for dog-ear repair, the basic technique is to remove the triangle of tissue that is causing the dog-ear or pucker. There are several methods for doing this. If the surgeon remembers to triangulate the excess tissue, the dog-ear can be satisfactorily corrected with greater ease. With practice, the surgeon can even curve the dog-ear repair into relaxed skin tension lines, to better hide the closure and avoid absolute straight lines. Outlined below are five methods for dog-ear repair.

Method 1: This method is the classic bilateral dog-ear repair. It is simple and easily done. The surgeon first elevates a "tent" of tissue with a skin hook (see Figure 28A). An incision is then made along one side (Figure 28B); be sure to extend it to the end of the tent. Next, the resulting triangle of skin is pulled over the suture line (Figure 28C) and excised. The wound is closed with simple interrupted stitches (Figure 28D).

Figure 28
Bilateral dog-ear repair

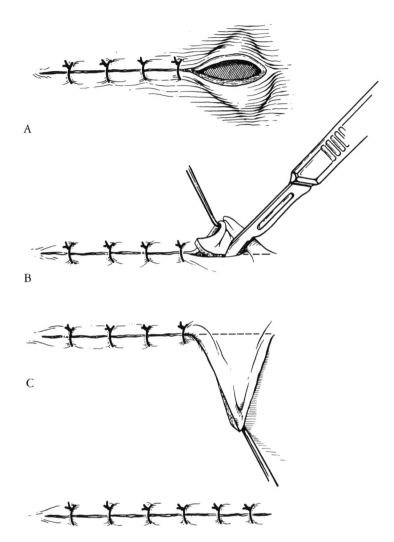

A

B

C

D

Method 2: This method is the unilateral dog-ear repair. When a one-sided dog-ear exists after closure of a wound, it can be removed using the "hockey-stick" closure. A tent of tissue is raised with a skin hook (Figure 29A), and one side is incised to the end of the tent (Figure 29B). The remaining triangle of tissue is pulled over the incision and excised (Figure 29C). The wound is closed with interrupted stitches (Figure 29D).

Figure 29
Unilateral dog-ear repair
(hockey stick)

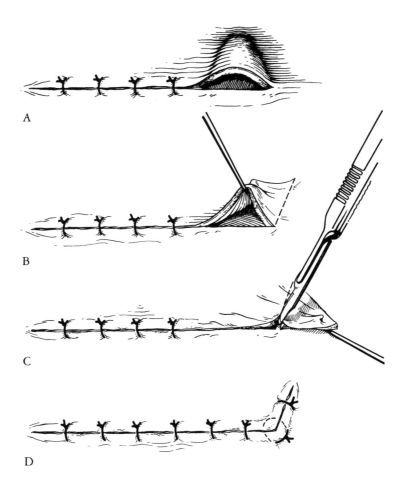

A

B

C

D

Method 3: This simple method is used to repair small dog-ears. To perform it, the surgeon simply extends the original incision by making an elliptical incision around the dog-ear in contiguity with the original suture line (Figure 30A).

Method 4: This method is a variation of method 3, only the surgeon uses an M-plasty (a discussion of M-plasty can be found under Basic Variations of the Fusiform Excision (Ellipse), which appears in the next section of this chapter) to shorten the length of the dog-ear repair (Figure 30B).

Method 5: Like method 3, this technique involves simply making a second ellipse. This method is used when a bulky dog-ear is left, requiring that the second ellipse be made perpendicular to the incision line (Figure 30C).

**EXERCISE 18:
BILATERAL DOG-EAR
REPAIR**

1. Examine your work thus far for possible dog-ears, or make an oval excision and close it with one interrupted stitch in the center of the oval, creating a bilateral dog-ear.
2. Using method 1 (see Figure 28), remove the dog-ear by triangulating the excess tissue that forms it.
3. Repeat this method until you are comfortable with it.

Exercises 22 and 24 deal with method 4, the M-plasty; please delay practicing this method until the exercises for it are introduced.

**EXERCISE 19:
UNILATERAL DOG-
EAR REPAIR**

1. Excise a semicircle.
2. Begin at one apex of your excision and close, taking bites equidistant from the apex on each side of the defect. Continue this procedure, creating a unilateral dog-ear.
3. Refer to Figure 29B. Grasp the dog-ear with a skin hook, creating a tent.
4. Make an incision (see Figure 29B), extending it to the end of the tent.
5. Release the triangle of tissue created by the initial incision. Cut along the base of this triangle (see Figure 29C).
6. Remove the triangle of tissue, thus creating a curved or "hockey-stick" dog-ear repair.
7. Close this incision by placing a three-point corner (tip) stitch, as outlined in Exercise 10 and Figure 19.
8. Repeat this exercise until you feel comfortable with this method of dog-ear repair.

Figure 30
Variations of dog-ear
repair

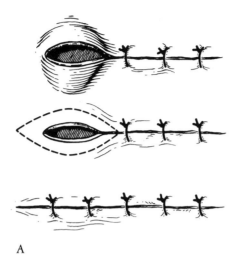

A

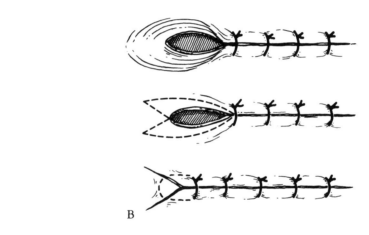

B

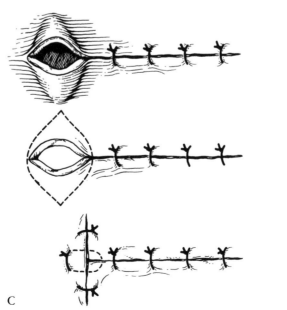

C

Basic Variations of the Fusiform Excision (Ellipse)

CURVING THE ELLIPSE

In cutaneous surgery, it is often necessary to curve the line of closure to match or to parallel relaxed skin tension lines. With careful planning, this can easily be accomplished by creating wounds of unequal length. In planning and diagramming your ellipse, one side of the ellipse is made shorter than the opposite side, and the ellipse is closed using the rule of halves. As illustrated in Figure 31, this method curves the ellipse to match skin tension lines. Figure 31A shows that the shorter side of the excision can even be curved to allow accentuation, or a greater curve, of the closure. Figure 31B illustrates the rule of halves.

EXERCISE 20: CURVING THE ELLIPSE

1. Draw an ellipse with one side straighter and shorter than the other, as shown in Figure 31A.
2. Excise the ellipse, and undermine.
3. Using the rule of halves, close the center of each side of the ellipse with an interrupted stitch as diagrammed in Figure 31B.
4. Follow the rule of halves to finish the closure, using interrupted stitches.

Figure 31
(A) Curving the ellipse
and (B) the rule of
halves

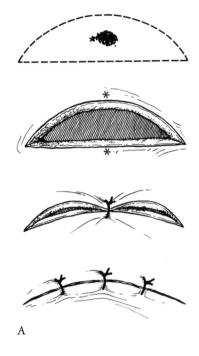

A

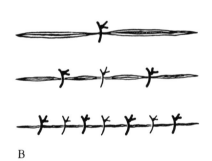

B

LAZY S EXCISION

The basic principle of camouflaging a scar in cutaneous surgery is to break up a straight line. You just learned how to curve a line. The lazy S excision is another way to break up a straight line, by making two curves. As illustrated in Figure 32, the excision is diagrammed in a fashion that will yield two curves upon closure. By closing these two curves of the lazy S, as shown in Figure 32, the wound can be closed without the formation of dog-ears.

EXERCISE 21: LAZY S EXCISION

1. Draw a small hypothetical lesion on the pig's foot and outline the lazy S excision, as shown in Figure 32.

2. Make the incision, carefully remove tissue, and undermine.

3. Using two skin hooks or skin hook and forceps, grasp the lazy S excision at the points marked with an asterisk in Figure 32, and cross your hands. This will show you where to place the initial stitch to align the lazy S closure.

4. Place an interrupted stitch at the meeting of the points that you have grasped. This should align the closure, which can then be finished with whatever stitch you prefer.

Figure 32
Lazy S

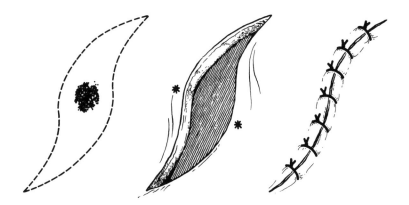

M-PLASTY (CROWN CLOSURE)

The M-plasty is the third basic variation of the ellipse. The M-plasty, sometimes called the crown closure, is invaluable to the cutaneous surgeon. It is essentially a length-shortening maneuver. Theoretically, by making an M-plasty, the total length of the ellipse can be shortened by one-fourth. The M-plasty can also be used to remove a dog-ear or to shorten the area of a flap. Its usefulness in these functions will be demonstrated in Chapter 2 during the discussion of more advanced flaps.

Figure 33 illustrates the ideal geometry for an M-plasty, and reemphasizes the importance of the 30-degree angle in the geometry of skin closure. The figure shows the creation of two 30-degree angles when the M is made. By performing an M-plasty at one end of the incision, the length of the scar can be shortened by one-fourth. When beginning an M-plasty, always diagram the entire fusiform excision first, before drawing the M. This will yield a better understanding of the geometry of this closure.

EXERCISE 22: M-PLASTY

1. Referring to Figure 33, draw an ellipse on the pig's foot and a line bisecting each apex of the ellipse; measure this line for later reference.
2. Three-fourths of the distance along this line, make a dot.
3. Draw a straight line from the dot to each side of the ellipse, creating two 30-degree angles and outlining the M.
4. Make your incision, cutting the tips of the M very carefully with scissors, and undermine. Make sure to undermine the tips of the M.
5. Place an initial interrupted stitch, using the rule of halves. This will help align the M for closure. Place sutures as needed to remove tension from the tip of the M. Next, close the tip of the M using a three-point corner (tip) stitch, as outlined in Exercise 10 and Figure 19. Begin the stitch 2 mm before the point of the M, to pull the M slightly forward upon completion of the stitch.
6. Finish suturing in any stitch desired.
7. Prove to yourself by measuring the closed wound that you have eliminated one-fourth of the original length of the ellipse by performing an M-plasty.

Figure 33
M-plasty

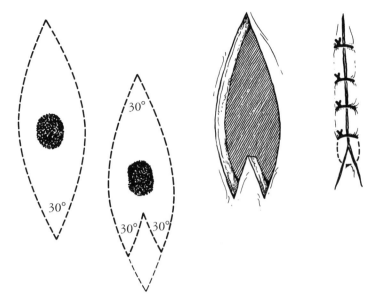

**DOUBLE OR
BILATERAL M-PLASTY**

If one **M**-plasty can conserve the length of the tissue by one-fourth, then two can conserve more. Where possible, a double **M**-plasty will shorten the length of the incision by approximately one-half. It is outlined and performed in a fashion similar to that of the single **M**-plasty, with the same geometry, only an **M** is made at both ends of the ellipse (Figure 34).

**EXERCISE 23: DOUBLE
M-PLASTY**

1. Draw an ellipse, as in Exercise 3.
2. Draw a line bisecting each apex of the ellipse and measure it, as in Exercise 22. Divide this line into halves and then into fourths with dots.
3. From one of the end dots, draw two lines to the sides of the ellipse, producing 30-degree angles as in Exercise 22. Repeat this procedure at the other end of the ellipse.
4. Carefully cut the ellipse and the **M**-plasties, and undermine.
5. Place an interrupted stitch at the dot at the midportion of the ellipse, to align both ends of the **M**-plasty (according to the rule of halves). Close each tip using a three-point corner (tip) stitch, as previously described and performed.
6. Finish your closure.
7. Prove to yourself by measuring that you have shortened the total length of the ellipse by about one-half.

Figure 34
Double M-plasty

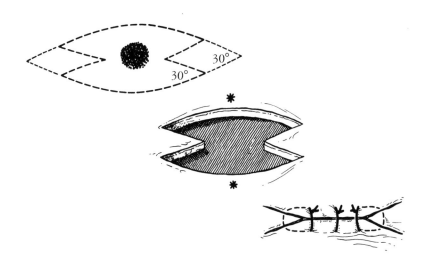

EXERCISE 24: M-PLASTY FOR DOG-EAR REPAIR

1. Refer to Figure 35 and Dog-ear Repair, method 4 (discussed previously in this chapter), for this exercise.

2. Make a circular or oval lesion and place a suture in the middle of it, creating two bilateral dog-ears.

3. Draw margins for an elliptical excision around one of the dog-ears, as shown in Figure 30.

4. Cut one-half the distance along each side of the ellipse, and undermine. This frees an arrow-shaped double triangle of tissue.

5. Beginning at the apex of the arrow, excise two triangles of excess skin, as shown in Figure 35.

6. Close by placing a three-point corner (tip) stitch, in order to gain practice using this technique.

7. Repeat this process to correct the dog-ear on the opposite side of the wound.

Figure 35
Steps in doing an M-plasty for a dog-ear repair

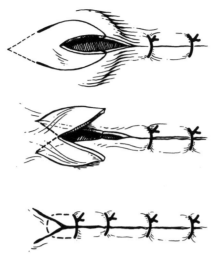

Practice Tests

TEST 1

1. Make a 0.5- × 1.0-cm hypothetical lesion.
2. Diagram a fusiform excision along the long axis of the lesion.
3. Excise the lesion using blunt dissection, undermining as you go.
4. Place a vertical mattress stitch in the center of the defect. Using the rule of halves, finish the closure by placing vertical mattress stitches alternating with simple interrupted stitches.

TEST 2

1. Make a lesion and excise it, as described in Test 1. Be sure to undermine.
2. Place interrupted subcutaneous stitches, alternating the placement of the knots (first with knot up and then with knot down). Remember to pull parallel to the axis of the wound when tying the knots.
3. Close the center of the wound with an interrupted stitch, using the rule of halves. Cut one end of the suture short and one end long.
4. Beginning on the left side of the excision, close to the midline, using a running locked stitch. To finish the stitch, tie to the end of suture left long.
5. Beginning on the right side of the excision, close using a running horizontal mattress stitch. Again, finish by tying to a loose end of the initial stitch placed in the middle of the closure.

TEST 3

1. Make a long, narrow ellipse, and undermine.
2. Place several subcutaneous interrupted stitches with the knots down.
3. Close using a running subcuticular stitch. Remember to exit periodically along the length of the wound to ensure ease of suture removal.
4. Close any small open areas of the excision or areas that are uneven in height using interrupted epicuticular stitches.

TEST 4

1. Make a lesion as in Test 1, excise it, and undermine.
2. Place a central horizontal mattress "stay" suture, using the rule of halves.
3. Close the lesion with several interrupted and/or vertical mattress stitches.
4. Remove the horizontal mattress stitch.

TEST 5

1. Make a 0.5- × 1.0-cm hypothetical lesion.
2. Outline an ellipse that curves the excision, mimicking skin tension lines.

3. Excise the lesion, and undermine.

4. Close, using a central vertical mattress stitch. Remember the rule of halves.

5. Continue using the rule of halves to close the remaining curved ellipse.

TEST 6

1. Diagram a fusiform excision, as described in Test 1.

2. Using your pen or gentian violet, modify each end of the excision to produce a bilateral **M**-plasty, maintaining 30-degree angles in the apices of each.

3. Excise it, and undermine.

4. Place a subcutaneous stitch, with the knot down, in the center of the excision. Tie the knot by pulling parallel to the axis of the wound, aligning both ends of the **M**-plasty for closure.

5. Place interrupted stitches as needed to remove tension from the tips of the **M**-plasty.

6. Close each **M**-plasty using a three-point corner (tip) stitch, remembering to pull the tip of the **M** slightly forward with the closure. Also, remember to maintain a uniform plane (middermal) in the skin edges and tip of the **M**.

TEST 7

1. Diagram and make a fusiform excision with sides of unequal lengths, as in Test 5.

2. Begin at the left side of the lesion and sew the extra tissue on the long arc of the wound to the right side, placing interrupted stitches with bites equidistant from the left apex.

3. Remove the unilateral dog-ear created in Step 1, using the hockey-stick method of dog-ear repair. Remember to triangulate the excess skin, and make the initial incision long enough to reach the end of the tent of tissue created by pulling up on the dog-ear with a skin hook.

4. Close the hockey-stick repair using a three-point corner (tip) stitch.

TEST 8

1. Remove a 1.0- × 1.5-cm oval of tissue.

2. Place an interrupted stitch in the center of the oval, creating bilateral dog-ears on each side.

3. Remove the dog-ear from the right side in the classic fashion by extending the line of incision. This frees a triangle of tissue for removal.

Remember to make your initial incision long enough, extending to the end of the tent raised by pulling up with a skin hook.

4. Remove the dog-ear from the left side by shortening the incision line with an **M**-plasty. This procedure will remove two small triangles of tissue. Close, using any method with which you feel comfortable.

2 Advanced Techniques: Local Flaps

Classification of Flaps

Key Techniques
 Undermining
 Corner Stitch
 Dog-Ear Repair
 Closing Wounds of Unequal Length
 Methods of Tension Release

Advancement Flaps
 Advanced Variations on the Ellipse
  Half-Ellipse (T Closure)
  Wedge Excision
  Island Advancement
 Single Advancement Flap (U-Plasty)
 Double Advancement Flap (H-Plasty)
 V-Y-Plasty
 Y-V-Plasty
 O-T- or T-Plasty

Rotation Flaps
 Single Rotation Flap: Triangular Defect
 Single Rotation Flap: Circular Defect
 Double Rotation Flap (O-Z)

Transposition Flaps
 Single Transposition Flap
 Bilobe Transposition Flap
 Rhombic Flap
 Variations of the Rhombic: Webster 30-Degree Angle Flap
 Z-Plasty

Practice Tests

Once you have mastered the basic techniques of cutaneous surgery, it is not difficult to advance to more complicated surgical techniques, such as flaps and grafts. This chapter emphasizes flaps; a discussion of grafts follows in Chapter 3. A **flap** is defined as the movement of an adjacent combination of skin and subcutaneous tissue from one location to another, with its vascular supply intact. The flap contrasts with the skin **graft,** which is the movement of a piece of tissue, usually from a distant site on the body, without its own vascular network. The graft, therefore, depends on several factors of the recipient site to form its own neovascular bed.

Critical to the performance of good flap surgery, as to the performance of any good cutaneous surgery, is a thorough understanding of the basics: (1) advancement of tissue, (2) rotation of tissue, and (3) transposition of tissue. These are the three basic methods of moving tissue from one body site to another. Some definitions relating to flap design and movement follow. The **primary defect** is the original wound to be closed. The **secondary defect** is the wound created by moving tissue from one site to another, in order to close the primary defect. With good flap design, the secondary defect is created in an area of loose tissue that can be easily approximated. In the case of very large flaps, the secondary defect may need to be closed with a graft. The **primary motion** of the flap is the motion or stress placed on it in order to close the primary defect. The **secondary motion** of the flap is the motion or stress placed on the tissue surrounding the primary defect by the performance of the primary motion. Therefore, there is a combination of stresses, primary and secondary, that occurs with the movement of a flap.

The final stresses on tissue, and therefore, on skin lines and surrounding fixed structures (e.g., eyelids or orifices) are the summation of the primary and secondary motions, or **vector forces,** on the flap. Therefore, it is important not only to fit the final suture lines of the flap within appropriate cosmetic skin lines, but also to understand the stresses that are placed on surrounding tissue by the primary and secondary motion used in creating the closure.

Skin has two important properties that enable tissue movement. These are **elasticity** and **movability. Elasticity** refers to the ability of skin to stretch. Skin on different areas of the body has differing amounts of elasticity. Cheek skin, for example, is very elastic, whereas scalp skin is not. **Movability** refers to the ability of skin to be moved from one site to another, and is unrelated to elasticity. For example, temple skin is less movable than cheek skin, although they are similar in elasticity.

Classification of Flaps

Flaps have several different classifications, depending on the textbook source and the complexity of the flap. Most texts begin by dividing flaps according to **anatomic location** (i.e., distant versus local flaps). **Distant flaps** usually involve movement of tissue from a distant source to repair a defect; an example would be movement of a large myocutaneous flap or free flap. **Local flaps** involve movement of tissue adjacent to the defect to cover it. Flaps are also classified by their **blood supply.** The two terms used in this classification are axial pattern flaps and random pattern flaps. **Axial pattern flaps** are designed to be based upon a named artery. **Random pattern flaps** are designed to take advantage of the cutaneous perforating vasculature and subdermal and dermal vascular plexuses; they are not necessarily based on a named artery. The basic cutaneous flaps described in this atlas are random pattern local flaps. Most axial pattern flaps have some random pattern to them, especially at the tip of the flap. Axial pattern and distant flaps are far beyond the scope and intent of this book. Another concept in flap surgery is **flap delay.** When attempting to obtain a greater length-to-width ratio in a flap, it may be necessary to cut the flap and then replace it on its original vascular bed, leaving it there for a period greater than a week before proceeding with the remaining flap surgery. This technique allows for better random vascularization of the tip of the flap before it is moved. This is called a **delayed flap.**

A classification of local random pattern flaps appears in Table 1. I have found this to be a very useful classification for basic flaps and basic tissue movement. Table 1 shows the three basic types of random pattern local flaps: advancement, rotation, and transposition. **Advancement**

Table 1. Local random pattern flaps

Advancement flaps	Rotation flaps	Transposition flaps
Island pedicle advancement	Single rotation	Single transposition
Single advancement (**U**-plasty)	Double rotation (**O-Z**)	Double transposition (bilobe)
Double advancement (**H**-plasty)	Multiple rotations	Rhombic and variations
Y-V, V-Y		**Z**-plasty
T-plasty		

flaps are flaps that involve advancement of local tissue to cover a primary defect. They are the simplest and easiest flaps to perform. The most basic advancement flap is the simple fusiform excision, but several different types of advancement flaps will be illustrated. **Rotation flaps** are flaps that are rotated around a pivot point to close a primary defect. There are very few defects where a rotation flap is not one of the closure options. They are conceptually somewhat more difficult than advancement flaps, but can be performed with rewarding results. **Transposition flaps** are flaps that are lifted and transposed around a pivot point in order to cover a primary defect. They are perhaps the most exciting flaps to perform, since they require the actual transposition, or lifting, of tissue from one site to another. Their geometry and design are more critical and difficult than the geometry and design of advancement or rotation flaps. As Table 1 shows, there are several different methods of advancing, rotating, or transposing tissue. These methods will form the crux of this chapter. We will not deal with interpolation flaps, island flaps, myocutaneous flaps, or free flaps with microvascular anastomosis as these are out of the realm of basic cutaneous surgery.

With an understanding of these basic terms and classifications, the student can begin to plan the flap. Each defect that is created will have several closure options. An understanding of the final geometry of the wound closure and of the stresses it places on adjacent skin enables the surgeon to pick the most appropriate flap for the location and point in time. A basic principle of all cutaneous surgery is to use the easiest and simplest technique necessary to repair any defect. For example, it is neither necessary nor appropriate to transpose a rhombic flap into a small defect that could be closed by a simple elliptical excision.

You should consider several things when planning a flap:

1. One advantage of a flap is that the surgeon can move adjacent skin of similar texture, color, and thickness into a defect while maintaining the skin's own blood supply. Therefore, when planning a flap, the properties of adjacent skin should always be kept in mind.

2. It is important not to be rigid in planning a flap. Often, after undermining and "playing" with the tissue, it becomes evident that the flap originally planned might not be the best. As one performs the flap, it may also become evident that the fine points of the flap (e.g., the placement of the Burrow's triangle) might best be done in a method other than the one initially planned.

3. When possible, even with random pattern flaps, the flap should be based near a major blood vessel or a branch thereof. Therefore, a knowledge of vascular anatomy is important in the design of flaps.

4. In general, the length of a flap should not be more than three times the width at its base. This gives the best chance of survival to the tip of the flap without compromising blood supply at the base of the flap. The concept of flap delay is important for larger flaps.

5. Once a flap is planned, cut, and moved into place, the basic surgical techniques and careful tissue handling that you have already learned are essential. A fine line scar can be obtained with a large flap as easily as it can with a simple ellipse.

6. The sutures should be placed from the flap to adjacent skin. Sutures should not be placed across the base of the flap. Every attempt should be made to widen the base of the flap and thus not compromise its blood supply.

7. Hemostasis prior to suturing the flap is essential, as hematoma is one of the leading causes of failure of flaps to survive.

8. It is important for the surgeon to realize, and to counsel his or her patient, that sensation and sweating are lost immediately after tissue transfer but may return after an interval of months to years.

Key Techniques

There are several basic techniques that are critical to flap surgery. These key techniques are reviewed below. The first three were covered in detail in Chapter 1, and the student should return there to review these techniques before proceeding. A critical discussion of wounds of unequal length and methods of tension release will follow the review of basic techniques.

UNDERMINING

Undermining is discussed in Chapter 1. You should review Exercise 5 for this technique before going any further, as undermining is critical to the movement of flap tissue. The plane of undermining will vary, depending on the depth of the tissue to be moved. Remember that the random pattern flap maintains its own blood supply from the subcutaneous and dermal plexus arterial network. Because of this, undermining should always be done at a minimum level of subcutaneous fat, so as not to interfere with these structures; depth will vary with anatomic location, however. Generally, it is difficult to undermine too much. Usually, the more the surgeon undermines, the less tension there will be on wound edges, and the easier it will be to take advantage of the movability and elasticity of tissue. Undermining can be blunt or sharp. I prefer blunt undermining, using a skin hook held like a pencil. In this way, your fourth and fifth fingers are free to "feel" the tip of the scissors while undermining. This allows the surgeon to maintain a uniform depth of undermining, and to know exactly where the tips of the instrument that is being used to undermine are. We will practice undermining throughout this section, as this technique is key to tissue movement.

CORNER STITCH

The three-point and four-point corner (tip) stitches are essential to good flap surgery. Exercises 10 and 12 should be reviewed and their methods well understood before proceeding further. Figures 19 and 22 are also relevant.

DOG-EAR REPAIR

The dog-ear repair is essential to good cutaneous surgery. Review the dog-ear repair with Exercises 18, 19, and 24. The most important aspect of the dog-ear repair is the removal of a triangle of tissue. This can be done in any one of a number of ways as is illustrated in Figures 28–30, and 35. The most common error in removing a dog-ear is not making the initial incision (initial side of the triangle of tissue to be removed) long enough. It is possible to curve the dog-ear repair to fit skin lines; this can be done by curving the initial incision line. A technical point important in the cutting of all flaps is that the best cut can often be made by first scoring the skin with the scalpel blade. A pair of sharp scissors, either straight or curved, can then be used to exactly cut the underlying dermis and subcutaneous tissue in the desired fashion.

Make sure that you are very facile with the dog-ear repair before continuing.

CLOSING WOUNDS OF UNEQUAL LENGTH

One method of closing wounds of unequal length has already been discussed in the explanation of how to curve an ellipse, found in Exercise 20 and Figure 31 in Chapter 1. When a flap is created, a wound of unequal length often remains that must be closed. There are several ways to do this. The three most common are illustrated in Figure 36. The first method (Figure 36A) uses the rule of halves as shown in Exercise 20. In this method, the extra tissue on one side of the closure is distributed throughout the length of the closure. The second method shown is removal of a triangle of tissue on the longer side of the wound, thus shortening it. Some people refer to this as a Burrow's triangle. It is essentially the removal of a dog-ear. Although the classic diagrams for flaps that

Figure 36
Closing wounds of
unequal length

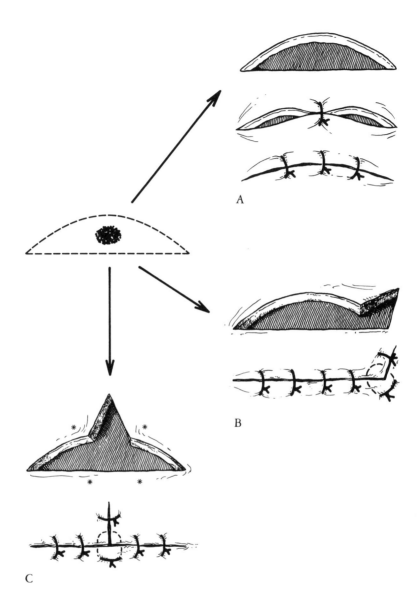

A

B

C

are seen in surgery texts often place the Burrow's triangle at the distal portion of the closure (Figure 36B), this is not always necessary nor indicated. The Burrow's triangle or triangle of tissue may be removed anywhere along the longer side of the wound. In Figure 36C, the triangle is in the middle of the longer side. After removal of the triangle, a four-point corner (tip) stitch is used to close.

EXERCISE 25:
CLOSING WOUNDS OF
UNEQUAL LENGTH

1. Create a wound of unequal length, as diagrammed in Figure 36.
2. First, close this wound using the rule of halves. Remember, the principle is to distribute the extra length of the top part of the wound throughout the entire length of the closure. Note that this technique curves the final suture line.
3. Now, remove the stitches from the first closure. Beginning at the left end of the wound, close, forcing the extra tissue in the longer arc of the wound to the right. This will create a bunching of tissue at the distal end of the wound. Remove this as diagrammed in Figure 36B, using the techniques of the unilateral dog-ear repair. The first incision to be made is the line furthest to the right in the diagram. This allows the surgeon to drape a triangle of skin over the initial incision, allowing for removal of the precise amount of "excess" skin in the triangle. Proceed with suturing, using a three-point corner (tip) stitch (illustrated by the dotted line in Figure 36).
4. Make an excision, creating wounds of unequal length, as in step 1. Close the wound as illustrated in Figure 36C by removing a triangle in the midportion of the long arc. It is often helpful to put an interrupted stitch at the point near the asterisks in the diagram, to help align the closure and indicate how much of a triangle should be removed. Then proceed with the closure, using the four-point corner (tip) stitch, as diagrammed by the dotted line in Figure 36C.
5. Repeat all of these closures until you become very facile with them. Remember that the triangle can be removed anywhere along the long side of the wound, thus shortening it and equalizing the lengths of the sides of the closure.

METHODS OF
TENSION RELEASE

No matter how well a flap is designed, the surgeon is often confronted with an unusual amount of tension on the wound. It is important to know several methods of relieving such tension. Illustrated in Figure 37 are three common methods of relieving tension employed in cutaneous surgery. The first (Figure 37A) employs a stay stitch, often a horizontal

Figure 37
Methods of tension
release

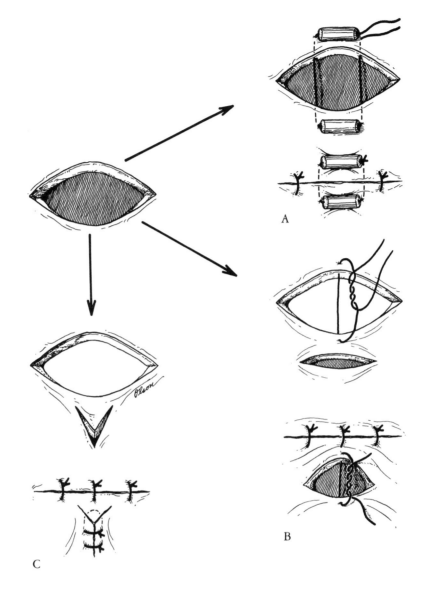

mattress stitch with or without bolsters, which serves to approximate tissue and align wound edges. When doing flap surgery, the stitch can often be placed as an initial stitch; it is surprising how the elasticity of the skin has adapted to this tension 5 to 10 minutes later, so that the remainder of the closure can be performed very easily, and the initial stay stitch can be removed. The second method (Figure 37B) is that of making another incision, adjacent to the initial wound and about two thirds its length. The initial wound is then closed, creating a second ellipse where the second incision was made. In this way, the great tension of the initial wound is shared between the two ellipses. The third method (Figure 37C) is making a V-shaped incision. The ellipse is then closed, and the V is sutured in place using a V-Y advancement flap, which will be discussed further in the section on advancement flaps included in this chapter.

A fourth method of tension release (not illustrated), which is often used on the scalp in making large flaps and/or scalp reductions, is the galea release incision. When the surgeon undermines on the scalp, the undermining occurs in the galea-periosteal plane. This leaves fibrous tissue (the galea) as the deepest portion of the flap. The tight, fibrous galea is the limiting factor in the movability of scalp flaps. By making an incision through the galea parallel to the axis of the closure, the surgeon can get more stretch for the closure. It is important not to make the galea incision too deep, as this compromises the dermal plexis blood supply to the flap.

EXERCISE 26: METHODS OF TENSION RELEASE

1. Make an ellipse with a 2 : 1 length-to-width ratio. This will produce a wound that should have some tension in the middle.
2. Use either the parallel or the V-incision method to release the tension, and proceed with the corresponding closure, as diagrammed in Figure 37.
3. Repeat this exercise, using whichever method you did not use in step 2.

Advancement Flaps

Because they are the simplest flaps to understand and perform, the discussion of flaps will begin with advancement flaps. The simplest advancement flap is the ellipse, introduced in Chapter 1. The ellipse, as you recall, is closed by bringing the two sides of the tissue together. Simple variations of the ellipse, such as curving the ellipse, the lazy S closure and the M-plasty, were all covered in Chapter 1. The discussion of advancement flaps will begin with advanced variations of the ellipse, including the half-ellipse, the wedge excision, and island advancement. Discussions of the single advancement flap (U-plasty), double advancement flap (H-plasty), V-Y- and Y-V-plasties, and O-T-plasty will follow.

ADVANCED VARIATIONS ON THE ELLIPSE

*Half-Ellipse (*T-Closure)

As illustrated in Figure 38, if an ellipse is halved, a triangular-shaped wound is left to be closed. Such wounds often result when performing an ellipse that abuts an orifice or crosses an important anatomic area, such as the angle of the mandible. These can be closed using a T-type closure, sometimes referred to as an A-T-closure. By extending lines A and B as shown in Figure 38, the wound can be closed in the shape of

Figure 38
Half-ellipse (T-closure)

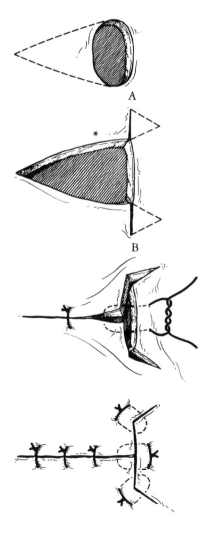

a geometric T. Because wounds of unequal length are created by performing the T-closure, it is often necessary to cut small Burrow's triangles when advancing the tissue.

EXERCISE 27: HALF-ELLIPSE (T-CLOSURE)

1. Diagram an ellipse with a 3 : 1 length-to-width ratio on the pig's foot.
2. Halve the ellipse with your marking pen, and shade one side.
3. Cut and remove the shaded area of the diagram.
4. Extend your incision along the line made to halve the ellipse.
5. Undermine.
6. Place your first stitch in the key area marked by the asterisks. This aligns the remainder of the closure.
7. Note the creation of wounds of unequal length, with an inner arc shorter than the outer arc. If necessary, remove triangles as diagrammed.
8. Proceed with the closure, using a four-point corner (tip) stitch in the center area of the T.
9. Congratulations! You have now performed your first flap.

Wedge Excision

Another variation of the ellipse, in fact a variation of the half-ellipse, is the through-and-through wedge excision. This excision might be performed on a lip or an ear. Illustrated in Figures 39 and 40 are techniques of lip wedge closure. This is a difficult technique to practice on a pig's foot. Practice of this technique should probably be done on foam or a cadaver. Therefore, no formal exercise concerning this technique will be presented.

After making sure of total tumor extirpation, the wedge excision follows in a step-wise progression, as illustrated in Figure 39. The vermilion border of the lip is first marked, using a small epicuticular stitch; this will help align the vermilion later in the closure. The excision is then made. I prefer beginning with a No. 11 blade and making a puncture through the lip at the apex of the wedge. The wedge is then removed, with the labial arteries isolated, clamped using a hemostat, and tied with suture ligatures. You will note in Figure 39B that the mucosal side of the wedge is smaller than the cutaneous side. Begin by first closing the mucosal surface, as illustrated in Figure 39C. I prefer using a running 5-0 chromic suture, making sure to evert mucosal surfaces. In this case,

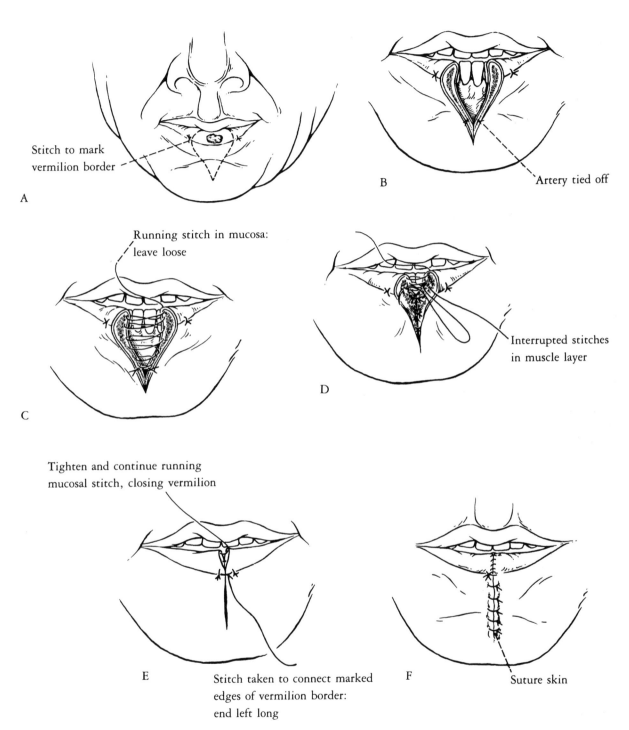

A — Stitch to mark vermilion border

B — Artery tied off

C — Running stitch in mucosa: leave loose

D — Interrupted stitches in muscle layer

E — Tighten and continue running mucosal stitch, closing vermilion

Stitch taken to connect marked edges of vermilion border: end left long

F — Suture skin

Figure 39
Wedge excision: lip

the stitch must be started from inside the mouth. A variation would be to place several interrupted canal stitches from the cutaneous side (inside) of the mucosa, as described in the section on variations of the horizontal mattress stitch in Chapter 1. Once the running stitch has closed the majority of the inner mucosal surface, it is left unfinished with a loose end. The interrupted, near-far, or purse-string closure of the orbicularis muscle that follows is illustrated in Figure 39D. Careful approximation of the muscle layer in closure is critical to prevent lip notching. The anterior ledge of the obicularis muscle must also be approximated. This is performed using 4-0 Dexon. Next, as illustrated in Figure 39E, the same 4-0 Dexon is used to place an interrupted stitch aligning the vermilion border at the areas that were previously marked. One end of the 4-0 Dexon is left long. The running mucosal stitch is then finished, closing the vermilion, as shown in Figure 39E. This is accomplished by tying the end of the running stitch to the loose long end of the vermilion stitch previously placed. The cutaneous surface is then sutured using interrupted stitches, usually with a monofilament suture, as illustrated in Figure 39F.

The cutaneous V of this wedge excision often extends well onto the chin. If the M-plasty is used to shorten the length of the incision, crossing the chin boundary can be prevented. The M-plasty adaptation of the lip wedge is illustrated in Figure 40.

Figure 40
Wedge excision: lip
wedge with M-plasty

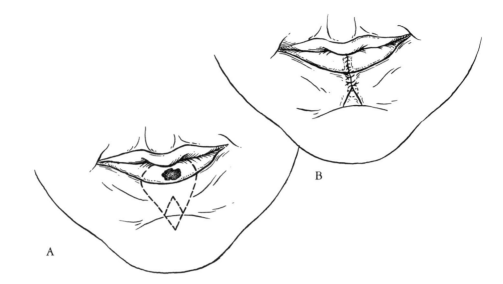

Island Advancement

The island advancement is the third advanced variation of the ellipse. It involves first diagramming an elliptical excision around a lesion as illustrated in Figure 41. The lesion is then removed, and the incisions for the ellipse are made. Instead of removing the normal tissue around the lesion, it is left in place. Undermining is carried out around the entire periphery of the incision lines, without undermining beneath the two islands of tissue (A and B in Figure 41). Still attached to their pedicle blood supply, these islands of tissue are advanced over the defect created by removing the lesion, and are sutured at the location marked by asterisks. Interrupted stitches can then be placed at what would be the apices of the ellipse as shown in Figure 41. This is an island pedicle advancement flap, useful on many areas of the body.

EXERCISE 28: ISLAND ADVANCEMENT FLAP

1. Draw a square hypothetical lesion, 5 mm × 10 mm.
2. Draw a fusiform excision with a 3.0–3.5 : 1.0 length-to-width ratio.
3. Incise and remove the hypothetical lesion only.
4. Incise the lines of the fusiform excision.
5. Using a skin hook and scissors, undermine **only** the periphery of the lesion as shown in Figure 41B, but be sure to undermine the entire periphery.
6. With islands of tissue A and B mobilized, place your first stitch in the areas marked by asterisks in Figure 41B, advancing the two islands of tissue together.
7. Close the apices of the ellipse with interrupted stitches, as shown in Figure 41C.
8. Finish the closure as desired.
9. Congratulations! You have just performed two **V-Y** advancement flaps (the island advancement variation of the fusiform excision).

Figure 41
Island advancement

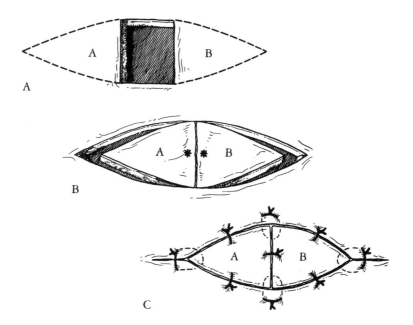

**SINGLE
ADVANCEMENT FLAP
(U-PLASTY)**

The single advancement flap is a very useful flap in certain anatomic sites, such as the eyebrow, sideburn area, and forehead. Perhaps its greatest usefulness is in helping understand some of the principles of tissue movement that are illustrated in Figure 42. Advancement is achieved by taking advantage of skin elasticity and by creating wounds of unequal lengths (see Figure 42): AC is greater than BC; DF is greater than EF. Classically, this flap is closed by excising Burrow's triangles laterally in the flap, thus equalizing the wounds of unequal lengths (AC′ = BC, DF′ = EF). As discussed earlier, it should be emphasized that it is not always necessary to remove the Burrow's triangle at the distal portion of the flap; it is done so here to illustrate the classic teaching of the advancement flap. The key stitch, which is placed first in the advancement flap, is placed at points 1 and 2 in Figure 42, thus closing the primary defect.

**EXERCISE 29: SINGLE
ADVANCEMENT FLAP
(U-PLASTY)**

1. Make a small, round defect about 3–4 in. from the amputated end of the pig's foot. This is a region where the skin is relatively loose. Then convert the round defect into a square, as shown in Figure 42.
2. Diagram the incisions to be made, as in Figure 42, extending the two sides toward the free end of the pig's foot. Shade in Burrow's triangles, as in Figure 42.
3. Make the incisions along the lines that you have marked.
4. Placing a skin hook at Point 1 in Figure 42, undermine the flap.
5. Using a skin hook as in the preceding step, pull the flap forward to join point 1 with point 2. You will see that a wound of unequal length has been created. Advance point 1, and place the key stitch.
6. Excise the triangles of tissue, as diagrammed in Figure 42, equalizing the wounds of unequal length. These triangles can be excised after placing the key stitch (as in an unequal dog-ear repair), or prior to placement of the stitch.
7. Once tension has been relieved, the corners of the flap are sutured using a corner (tip) stitch. The remaining flap is sutured as desired.

Figure 42
Single advancement flap
(U-plasty)

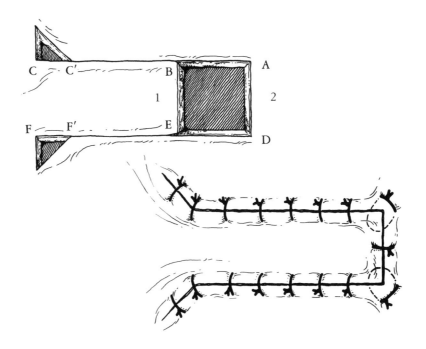

**DOUBLE
ADVANCEMENT FLAP
(H-PLASTY)**

As with the **M**-plasty, if one **U**-plasty or advancement flap is good, would two be better? The answer is often yes, especially in the case of lesions that are located directly in the eyebrow or sideburn. The basic principles of the closure are identical to those for the single advancement flap. The double advancement flap is diagrammed in Figure 43. Again, wounds of unequal length are created (AC + BD < CD; EG + FH < GH), which must be equalized during closure.

Figure 43
Double advancement
flap (H-plasty)

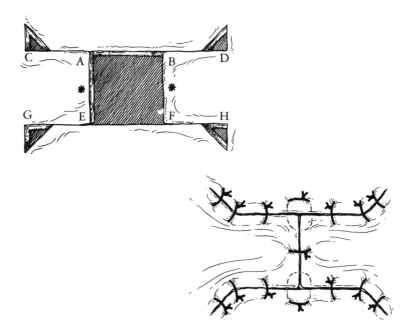

EXERCISE 30: DOUBLE ADVANCEMENT FLAP (H-PLASTY)

1. Create a square defect, as in Exercise 29.
2. Using a marker or gentian violet, outline the flap, as shown in Figure 44. Note that the sides of this flap need not be as long as for a single advancement flap.
3. Do not create Burrow's triangles yet, as you will close the wound of unequal length in various ways to illustrate how differently this closure can be accomplished.
4. Remove the defect, creating a square wound.
5. Cut and undermine both sides of the double advancement flap. Using your skin hook (placed at point 1) and your forceps (placed at point 2) advance the flap to make sure that it will freely join in the middle. If there is too much tension at the midpoint, extend your excision lines, undermine further, and then try to advance again. Place your key stitch between points 1 and 2 on Figure 44, and close the primary defect.
6. You now have two wounds of unequal length. Close the top left wound using the rule of halves. Close the top right wound by excising a Burrow's triangle distally along one side of the closure, and place a corner stitch, as diagrammed in Figure 44B. Equalize the length of the sides, and close the bottom arc by removing a triangle midway along that side instead of distally. Your key stitch will be a four-point corner (tip) stitch, as illustrated in Figure 44B.
7. Finish suturing the closure as you like.

Figure 44
Double advancement
flap (H-plasty)

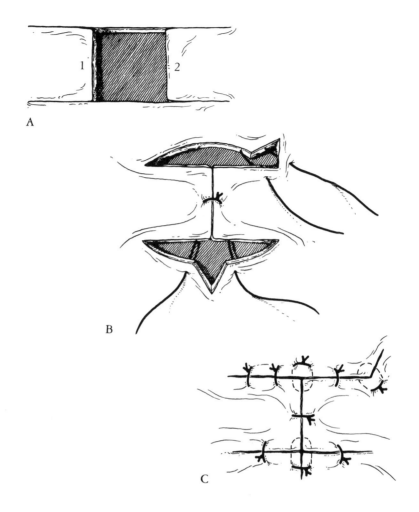

V-Y-PLASTY

The V-Y-plasty is a simple movement of tissue meant to ease tension in the direction of the open part of the V. This method of tension release was illustrated in Exercise 26. The V-Y-plasty can also be used to align cosmetically important areas and orifices that have been moved during previous surgery by raising an anatomic point. Figure 45 illustrates the V-Y-plasty. Exercises to practice this technique, as well as those for the Y-V-plasty, are difficult to do on a pig's foot and are better practiced on foam or cadaver skin.

EXERCISE 31: V-Y-PLASTY

1. Make a narrow V-incision in the pig's foot, as illustrated in Figure 45.
2. Placing a skin hook at point 1, lift and freely undermine the V.
3. Beginning at point 2, place two adjacent interrupted stitches. This will push point 1 in the direction of the arrow in Figure 45.
4. Place a three-point corner (tip) stitch, as illustrated.
5. Finish closing the V in the form of a Y. Note that the tip (point 1) has moved away from point 2.

Figure 45
V-Y-plasty

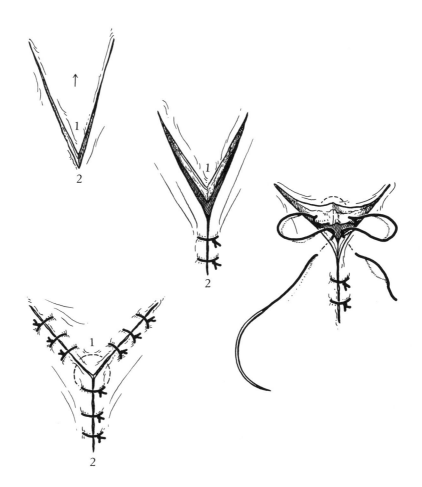

Y-V-PLASTY

Just as the **V-Y**-plasty may raise an anatomic point, the **Y-V**-plasty may lower one (such as an eyelid or lip), and relax tension, to some extent, in a lateral direction. It is performed in a manner opposite to that of the **V-Y**-plasty.

EXERCISE 32: Y-V-PLASTY

1. Make a **Y**-incision, as illustrated in Figure 46.
2. Using scissors and a skin hook, elevate point 1 and undermine. Also undermine the edges along the line marked 1–2.
3. Advance the tip (point 1) to meet point 2, and suture, using a three-point corner (tip) stitch.
4. Suture the remaining sides as desired.

Figure 46
Y-V-plasty

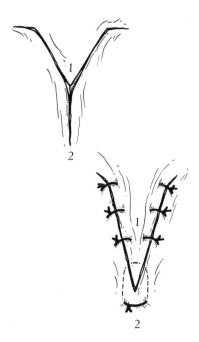

O-T- OR T-PLASTY

This closure is one of the most common used in cutaneous surgery. In Figure 47, the student can see that this closure can be accomplished from either a circle or a triangle. It is also possible to make the portion of the closure extending from the circle in Figure 47DE (dotted lines) an **M**-plasty, to shorten the length of that side. The **T**-plasty, like other flaps previously introduced, depends on the principle of creating and equalizing a wound of unequal length. The **T**-closure is a useful closure on any area of the body, particularly in or along hair-bearing areas where a portion of the closure can be hidden in the hairline.

EXERCISE 33: O-T- OR T-PLASTY

1. Excise a circular defect. Diagram a triangle, as shown in Figure 48. Shorten the triangle by performing an **M**-plasty. You now have completed an **M**-plasty dog-ear repair, as described in Figure 35.
2. Create the **T** by drawing the equivalent of the lines in Figure 48. DO NOT make the Burrow's triangles.
3. Using scissors and a skin hook, undermine the edges of the wound at the asterisks.
4. Cut along the marked lines to create the **T**-closure. The first stitch should be at the asterisks at the midpoint of the triangle in Figure 48, to begin the closure and align both the **M** and the wound edges. The key stitch has closed the primary defect.
5. You once again must close a wound of unequal length. This can be done by excising triangles, as you see in Figure 47, anywhere along the longer side. In this case, the extra length of the long edge will be distributed so that only one triangle needs to be excised. Beginning at the upper side of the wound, in Figure 48C, begin to suture this side of the **T**, using interrupted stitches equidistant from each side from the apex. This forces the majority of the loose tissue toward the distal end of the flap.
6. You have now created the equivalent of a dog-ear at the distal limb of the **T**. Excise this dog-ear in a hockey-stick fashion, as described in Chapter 1. By angling the incision along the lower side of the dog-ear, a triangle is created, which can be removed (Figure 48D).
7. Approximate the midportion of the **T** in the usual fashion, using a four-point corner (tip) stitch as diagrammed in Figure 48C.
8. Approximate the area where the dog-ear has been removed with a corner stitch. Finish the closure as desired.

Figure 47
O-T-plasty

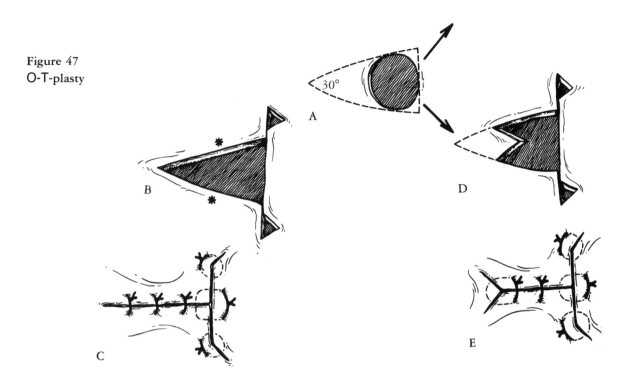

Figure 48
O-T-plasty with M-plasty

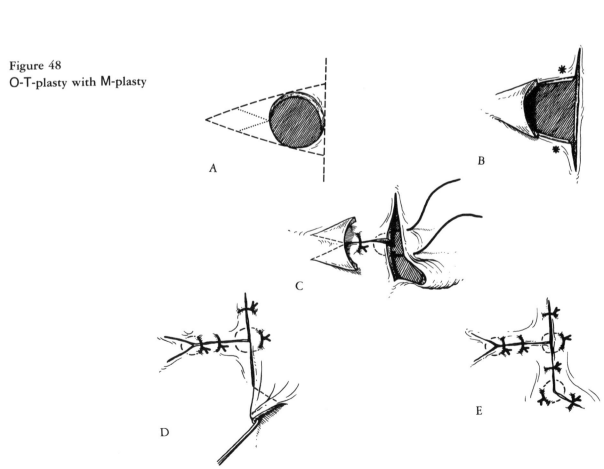

Rotation Flaps

The rotation flap is one of the most useful closures in cutaneous surgery. A thorough understanding of this flap will enable you to close circular defects in most anatomic sites. The rotation flap can be performed either as a single flap or as a combination of two, three, or sometimes four rotation flaps in the same closure (a pinwheel flap).

The principle behind the rotation flap is similar to that of advancement flaps. An arc of skin is cut and undermined, but is rotated instead of advanced, to cover the primary defect. This process creates a secondary defect, which must be closed using methods similar to those used for many advancement flaps. A wound of unequal length is created once the flap is rotated. Figure 49 diagrams the basic method for performing the rotation flap.

In Figure 49 the arc from A to D is cut. The distance from A to D is less than the distance from C to D. There are two ways to equalize the sides. As shown in Figure 49E, the longer, outer side can be shortened by removing a triangle of excess skin, as described previously. The second method, shown in Figure 49E, would require a back cut. This method in essence lengthens the shorter side in order to equalize the sides for closure. In general, the greater the area under the arc rotated, the greater the ease in closure and the less tension necessary to close the defect. The size of this area will vary depending on skin characteristics (movability and elasticity), anatomic location (e.g., orifices and hair-bearing skin), and desire to stay within cosmetic units and relaxed skin tension lines.

SINGLE ROTATION FLAP: TRIANGULAR DEFECT

With knowledge of the principles of the rotation flap outlined above and in Figure 49, the student can proceed with Exercise 34.

EXERCISE 34: ROTATION FLAP: TRIANGULAR DEFECT

1. Make a small circular defect near the amputated end of the pig's foot.
2. Convert this round defect into a triangle, as diagrammed in Figure 49, maintaining a 30-degree angle at the apex of the triangle.
3. Diagram the rotational arc AD as shown in Figure 49. In general, the greater the arc, the less tension placed on the primary defect closure, and the greater the diameter of the wound that can be closed.
4. Begin to cut the arc. Using a skin hook and elevating along line AB in Figure 49B, undermine and cut the entire arc. Either the undermining or the cutting of the arc can be performed first; experiment with each as you progress.

Figure 49
Rotation flap

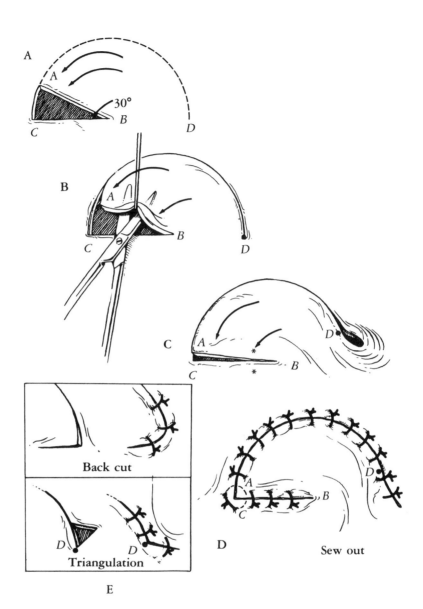

5. Elevate line AB, and rotate the arc to point C. The primary motion of this flap is in the direction of the arrows along line AB. Secondary motion will be opposite this direction, along line CB, with tension at point D.

6. Again, a wound of unequal length has been created. The inner side AD is shorter than the outer side CD. There are two ways to deal with this, the first being a back cut, and the second being a Burrow's triangle. In this exercise, we will perform a back cut.

7. Make a back cut at point D, as illustrated in Figure 49E. This will increase the length of the inner side of the flap.

8. The positioning of point A will vary, depending on the desired tissue movement. The entire triangle can be closed, maximizing the size of the secondary defect. The closure of the primary defect can be "shared" with the secondary defect by not completely rotating point A. This leaves a smaller secondary defect. Experiment with this concept by placing a temporary stitch at point A, without tying, and use this stitch to rotate the flap. Then remove the temporary suture, and suture the flap in place. The key stitch in the rotation flap will be a tacking stitch, joining the midpoint on line AB, with the midpoint of line BC, thus closing the primary defect. The exact position of this stitch can be determined using the temporary stitch.

9. Suture to remove tension from corners, placing the corner stitches as diagrammed in Figure 49D.

SINGLE ROTATION FLAP: CIRCULAR DEFECT

As shown in Figure 50, the rotation flap used to close a circular defect is based on the same principle as the flap for the triangular defect. The only real difference is that, in the case of the circular defect, the rotation of tissue produces a pucker or dog-ear of tissue in the area of the triangle shown in Figure 49. This dog-ear can be removed in one of several ways. The two easiest procedures use the techniques previously described for dog-ear removal or for the M-plasty, to shorten the length of the line created by removing the pucker that results from tissue rotation. Once the flap is cut, a wound with unequal sides is again created. It can be dealt with as shown in Figure 49, either by triangulating excess tissue from the long side, or by lengthening the inner side using a back cut. In the example given in Figure 50, the longer, outer side is shortened by excising a triangle of tissue. Remember, this triangle can be removed anywhere along the longer side of the wound; this principle is especially

Figure 50
Rotation flap: circular
defect

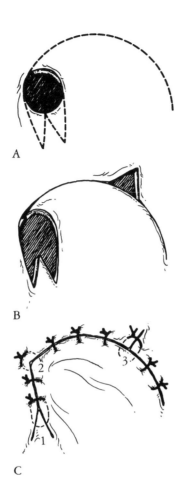

A

B

C

important when performing a flap near hair-bearing skin, such as the scalp or sideburn area, in order to hide the scar that results from removal of the triangle of tissue within the hair-bearing skin.

**EXERCISE 35:
ROTATION FLAP:
CIRCULAR DEFECT**

1. Make a circular defect as in Exercise 34, but do not triangulate it.

2. Proceed as in Exercise 34, drawing the arc of the rotation flap, cutting, and undermining the arc of tissue to be rotated.

3. Rotate the tissue as illustrated in Figure 49, placing the key stitch at the midpoint to close the primary defect. Remember the "sharing" concept described in Exercise 34. Experiment with a temporary suture placed as before to best determine the proper position of the key stitch.

4. You once again have created wounds of unequal length and also have created a dog-ear. Remove the dog-ear using an **M**-plasty, as illustrated in Figure 50A.

5. Equalize the lengths of the rotation flap sides by excising a triangle of tissue, as shown in Figure 50B. Remember that the triangle can be removed anywhere along the longer side, thus shortening it.

6. Place the remaining stitches, practicing the three-point corner (tip) stitch at points 1 and 2 and the four-point corner (tip) stitch at point 3.

**DOUBLE ROTATION
FLAP (O-Z)**

The **O-Z** double rotation flap has several uses. With an understanding of this flap and its final geometry, the surgeon can often place it very nicely within skin lines, especially in the forehead and temple areas. The **O-Z** double rotation flap is also useful for closing large scalp defects. Figure 51 illustrates the basic double rotation flap. The principles for diagramming and cutting this flap are the same as for the single rotation flap, only two arcs are made. Again, the wider the arc, the less tension will be placed on the closure, and the wider the diameter of the circle that can be closed. This is especially true for flaps used on the scalp, where the galea limits skin movability.

As shown in Figure 51, in some ways the double rotation flap is another variation of the ellipse, with only half of each side of the fusiform excision cut. As Figure 51 illustrates, wounds of unequal length are again created, and can be dealt with using the rule of halves (Figure 51C), shortening the long side by removing a triangle anywhere along it (Figures 51D and E), or by back cutting and lengthening the shorter side (Figures 51F and G).

Figure 51
O-Z rotation flap

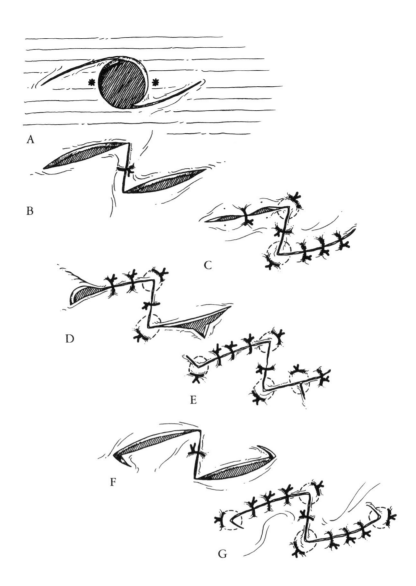

**EXERCISE 36: DOUBLE
ROTATION FLAP (O-Z)**

1. Cut a circular defect on the pig's foot.
2. Referring to Figure 51, diagram the arcs of the closure as shown. A good guideline for the arcs would be to draw them as the sides of what would be an ellipse, with a 3.5–4.0 : 1 length-to-width ratio.
3. Cut the arcs, and completely undermine the tissue to be rotated.
4. Using forceps and skin hook, rotate both sides of the flap into place to make sure they will join in the middle. If there is too much tension, undermine further, and extend the arcs of the flap.
5. Rotate the flaps, and place the key stitches at the points marked with asterisks in Figure 51A closing the primary defect. You have created two wounds of unequal length. You may deal with these in a number of ways.
6. Use a different method of triangulation to deal with each side of the flap, perhaps removing a triangle in the middle of the lower (right) side of the defect, and using a dog-ear repair at the distal portion of the upper (left) side, as shown in Figures 51D and E. Close as desired.
7. Repeat this procedure using another means of closure, such as those illustrated in Figures 51F and G.

Figure 52 illustrates three different multiple rotation flaps that are especially useful for large scalp and trunk defects.

Figure 52
Multiple rotation flaps

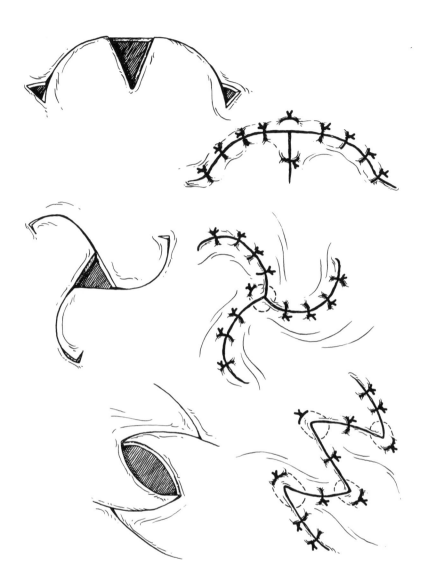

Transposition Flaps

Transposition flaps can be the most difficult, but also the most useful and rewarding flaps in cutaneous surgery. They involve the actual transposition (i.e., lifting and moving) of skin around a pivot point. The flap moves around that pivot point in an arc. A secondary defect is created by the flap's movement in this arc, which must be handled in a different way than the wound of unequal lengths that occurs in the creation of advancement and rotation flaps. The lines of force (i.e., the primary and secondary motions) are more subtle in transposition flaps, and must be fully understood to place these flaps within relaxed skin tension lines. Four basic transposition flaps will be discussed, beginning with the simplest and ending with the most complicated. Figure 53 illustrates the concepts of primary defect, secondary defect, pivot point, and arc of transposition.

The **primary defect,** by definition, is the original defect to be closed. The **secondary defect** is the defect created by the movement of tissue necessary to close the primary defect. This concept becomes important when closing a transposition flap because the key stitch, unlike that of the advancement and rotation flaps that was placed to close the primary defect, is placed to close the secondary defect. The **pivot point,** shown in Figure 53 at point A and at the asterisk, is the point about which a transposition flap moves. It is a critical point because the greatest line of tension on the flap originates from it. It is also the point from which the total length of the flap must be measured. For example, the length of the flap illustrated in Figure 53 would be measured from the pivot point to point B. A common mistake is to measure the length of the flap as the length of the primary defect (point C to point B in Figure 53). If this error is made, the flap transposed will be too short. The **arc of transposition** is the arc along which the flap moves. When a flap is transposed, a pucker or dog-ear is often created at the point marked C in Figure 53. Some surgeons prefer to leave the pucker to resolve or to be corrected in a secondary procedure. However, it can be removed primarily, using the methods for dog-ear excision. When this is done, the initial cut of the dog-ear removal must always widen the base of the flap.

There are several transposition flaps. The simplest is the single transposition flap. Although the rhombic and variations on the rhombic are also single transposition flaps, their geometry is more difficult to understand, they are named flaps, and they will be dealt with later in this chapter.

Figure 53
Transposition flap

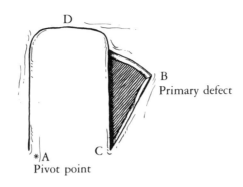

D

B
Primary defect

*A
Pivot point

C

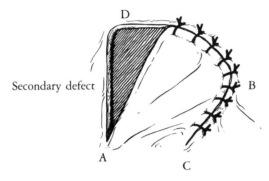

D

Secondary defect

B

A

C

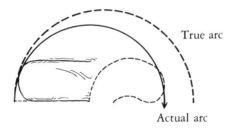

True arc

Actual arc

**SINGLE
TRANSPOSITION
FLAP**

Figure 54 shows the single transposition flap, illustrated as a nasolabial flap. Its principles are really very simple. It is usually performed in an anatomic site where the area of a primary defect is too great to close directly. Therefore, closure of that area is shared with tissue moved from an adjacent site, which has good color and texture match as well as the elasticity necessary to close the secondary defect. The nasolabial transposition flap is a classic example. Key to the flap is proper measuring. The length of the flap **must** be measured from the pivot point to the end of the defect. In Figure 54, this distance is line AB, with A being the pivot point. Therefore, line AB must equal line AD. The width of the single transposition flap is usually equal to the width of the defect. If there is some movability of tissue around the primary defect and/or lack of elasticity to easily close the secondary defect, the flap can be somewhat narrower than the width of the primary defect. If the defect is located on an important cosmetic area, such as below an eyelid or on a lip, it is best to make the flap slightly wider than the primary defect it will cover. When tissue is transposed, this allows the flap not only to fit, but also to actually push skin outward, as the secondary motion of the flap. This motion would be critical on an eyelid, for example, where incorrect, narrow, or short measurement could result in ectropion.

Another fine point to remember when performing the transposition flap is to excise and include the area shaded below point D in Figure 54 with the flap to be transposed. If the flap ended at point D with a curve as diagrammed, a dog-ear would result upon closure of the secondary defect. By excising this dog-ear and moving it with the flap, any error in measurement of the length of the flap can be overcome. The small triangle of tissue can then be excised after the flap has been transposed. Closure of the secondary defect can follow, without the necessity of dog-ear removal. Remember, the key stitch in a transposition flap closes the **secondary** defect, thus aligning the remainder of the closure.

**EXERCISE 37: SINGLE
TRANSPOSITION
FLAP**

1. Draw and excise a circular defect.
2. Find the area that will be the pivot point. This will be at approximately the midpoint of the base of the flap, and above it. Measure from this point to the far side of the defect, the equivalent of line AB in Figure 54. From point A, extending outward 60–90 degrees from the defect, draw the U-shaped transposition flap, measuring the length of line AB = AD.

Figure 54
Single transposition flap
(nasolabial)

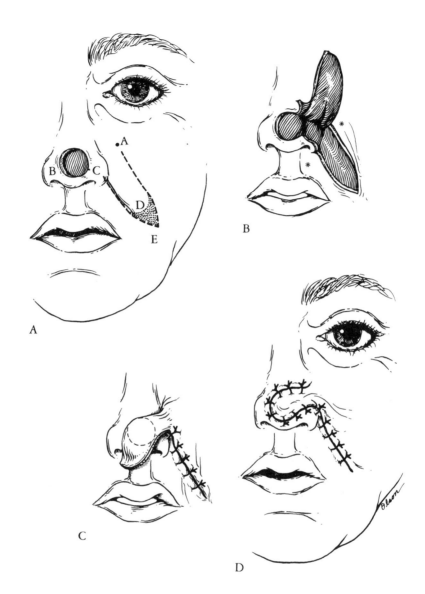

3. At point D on the pig's foot, draw a triangle as diagrammed by the shaded area in Figure 54.

4. Cut, undermine, and elevate the flap as shown in Figure 54B.

5. Place your key stitch at the point marked by the asterisks in Figure 54B, closing the secondary defect and aligning the flap. This stitch should be equidistant from point E and the asterisk on each side of the secondary defect.

6. Place the next stitch, aligning the sides of the flap.

7. Trim the excess length of the flap, and suture as shown in Figures 54C and D.

8. Finish suturing the closure in any way you desire.

BILOBE TRANSPOSITION FLAP

As with the **M**-plasty and the **O-Z** double rotation flap, if one transposition flap is good, would two be better? The bilobe flap illustrates the technique for performing two transposition flaps to repair one defect. Classically, this flap is drawn as in Figure 55. The volume under area A theoretically should be one-half to two-thirds of the volume of the primary defect (shaded area in Figure 55). The volume under area B should be one-half to two-thirds of that under A. In this way, by dividing the total volume of the shaded area between the volumes of areas A and B, this closure can be performed without distorting the primary defect. The pivot point is marked by a dot in the center of Figure 55. When measuring the bilobe flap, remember that the **vertical length** of this flap is measured from the pivot point. The **width** of each side is narrowed in order to achieve the volume reduction described above. Also, remember that the key stitch in a transposition flap closes the secondary defect; its placement is marked by asterisks in Figure 55, closing area B. Note that, as in the nasolabial single transposition flap, the length of area B can be increased with a triangle before cutting and transposing tissue (Figure 55). This gives extra length to that side of the flap, if needed, and removes the dog-ear that would have been created by closing the secondary defect. The bilobe transposition flap is often used when the primary defect is in inelastic skin, with skin that is more elastic nearby. The elastic skin, by means of a double transposition of tissue, can be used to indirectly close the inelastic primary defect. An example of this would be a nasal tip primary defect. The area represented by area B in Figure 55 ends up in the loose glabellar skin, allowing for easy closure of the primary defect. This is illustrated in Figure 56.

Figure 55
Bilobe flap

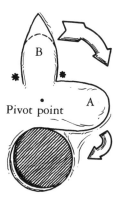

Figure 56
Bilobe flap showing
possible dog-ear

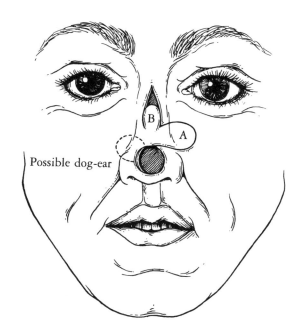

**EXERCISE 38: BILOBE
TRANSPOSITION
FLAP**

1. Draw a circular defect, as shown in Figure 55.
2. Following the principle that the volume beneath area A in Figure 55 should be two-thirds of the volume in the shaded area, draw arc A. Remember to extend the length of the flap to be transposed, so that when it is transposed about its pivot point (marked by the dot) it will be long enough.
3. Next, draw side B so that its volume is one-half to two-thirds the volume of side A. You can do this by decreasing the width of the flap but not the length. Remember the pivot point, and that the length of the sides of this flap must be equal from that point. Triangulate the tip of side B as shown in Figure 55.
4. Cut along the lines you have drawn, and widely undermine.
5. Elevate and transpose the tissue around the pivot point.
6. Close in the usual fashion, with the first stitch closing the secondary defect (shown under B in Figure 55), thereby aligning the entire flap. The second and third stitches should align and anchor the transposed tissue.
7. Close the flap as it covers the primary defect.
8. As in the single transposition flap, a dog-ear may result, as illustrated in Figure 56. This dog-ear can be left, or removed by widening the flap base. Redundant tissue is then removed, using a hockey-stick dog-ear repair.

RHOMBIC FLAP

The rhombic flap is most often used for the reconstruction of small to moderately large defects. The rhombic flap is based on the geometry of a rhombus (i.e., an equilateral parallelogram with oblique angles), as illustrated in Figure 57. It is perhaps the most difficult transposition flap to visualize geometrically.

For every rhombus, four closures are possible. These also are illustrated in Figure 57. By turning the rhombus 90 degrees and placing the lines in the opposite direction, a second four closures are created. Knowing the final geometry and vector forces of the flap will be important in deciding which of these closures will be most appropriate for the particular location of the incision. An example is shown in Figure 58. The first rhombic illustrated was incorrectly placed, and pulls down on the lower eyelid, producing ectropion. The correct placement of the second rhombic illustrated actually pushes up on the eyelid and prevents ectropion. Therefore, you should attempt to analyze the vector forces involved in

Figure 57
Rhombic flap

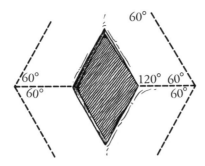

Figure 58
Rhombic flap: under eyelid

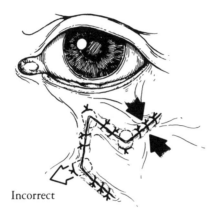

Incorrect

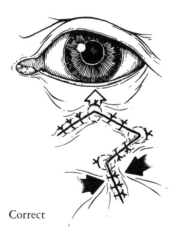

Correct

the flap as the rhombic flap is performed. The first person to describe this flap and whose name is often attached to it is Limberg; the Limberg flap is another name for the rhomboid.

The geometry of the rhombic flap is shown in Figure 59. The key, initial stitch is placed at the asterisks, closing the secondary defect. This will be the line of greatest tension on the closure, and also the line of secondary tissue motion. (Secondary tissue motion is the cause of the ectropion produced by the incorrect rhombic in Figure 58.) The final suture line can be visualized by covering lines AD and EF with a 3 × 5 card or your finger.

EXERCISE 39: RHOMBIC FLAP

1. Draw a parallelogram as in Figure 59, with the angles given in Figure 57. It should be drawn at the ankle of the pig's foot, as this is a difficult flap to close on inelastic skin.

2. Bisecting the 120-degree angle ADC, draw line DE. The length of this line should be equal to that of line BC.

3. With an angle of 60 degrees at point E, draw line EF (it should equal lines CD and DE).

4. Cut these lines, and undermine the entire flap, as well as the border of the parallelogram.

5. Using point A as the pivot point, grasp the tip of the flap at point E, and transpose the flap, matching point E′ with point C.

6. Place the key stitch at the asterisks along lines EF and DE to align the transposed tissue. The second stitch should be from side D′E′ to side BC, to anchor that portion of the flap. If these stitches are too difficult to place, review the geometry of the flap, and move on. Remember that the rhombic flap is difficult to perform on a pig's foot.

7. Close the remaining flap.

8. There may be a dog-ear at point A, which you should remove.

9. Practice performing this flap again, creating the flap from point B instead of point D, until you feel comfortable with its design and movement.

Figure 59
Performing the rhombic

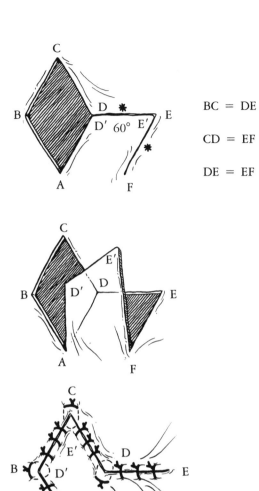

BC = DE

CD = EF

DE = EF

VARIATIONS OF THE RHOMBIC: WEBSTER 30-DEGREE ANGLE FLAP

The rhombic flap is based on the principle that the transposed flap is the same size and volume as the primary defect. In order for this flap to work, there must be enough loose tissue to close the secondary defect. Webster, using the principle of ideal angles of 30 degrees, created a flap where the tension on the closure of both the primary and secondary defects could be shared. He also realized that the dog-ear that was often created at point A of the rhombic flap was due to the fact that this point was at a 60-degree angle.

Review the angles of the parallelogram in Figure 57. They are the same as those in Figure 60A. Angle BCD equals angle BAD and is 60 degrees. As shown in Figure 60B, angle DEF (the tissue that will be transposed into angle BCD) is 30 degrees. By transposing a flap of half the volume of the primary defect into it, the closure of the primary defect is shared between the primary and the secondary defects.

Remember that a dog-ear is often produced at point A of the rhombic. In Figure 60B, by extending point A to create a 30-degree angle, this dog-ear can be removed in planning the flap. As discussed previously, the **M**-plasty is one way to shorten the length of a wound or remove a dog-ear. By using the geometry of an **M**-plasty, point A′ can be moved, as illustrated in Figure 60C, creating an **M**-plasty that shortens that side of the closure.

The Webster 30-degree angle flap is very useful and can be performed on almost any anatomic site. Its geometry and mechanics are much simpler than they look, once you understand the flap's principles. It also is a much easier flap to perform on inelastic skin, such as a pig's foot, since there is less tension on the closure of the secondary defect.

EXERCISE 40: WEBSTER 30-DEGREE ANGLE FLAP

1. Draw a parallelogram, as in Exercise 39.
2. Design the flap as pictured in Figure 60B, with line DE equal in length to line BC.
3. Creating a 30-degree angle at point E, draw line EF equal in length to line CD and line DE.
4. Extend point A to create a 30-degree angle at this end of the flap. Shorten the length of this end using the principles of the **M**-plasty, as diagrammed.
5. Cut the flap, and widely undermine both the flap and the parallelogram.

Figure 60
Variations on the rhombic—Webster 30-degree angle flap

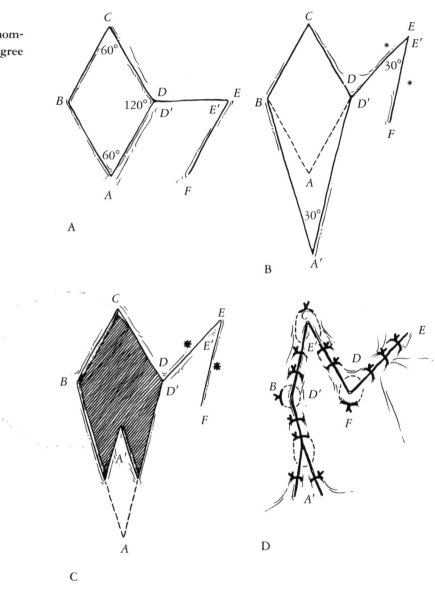

A

B

C

D

BC = DE

CD = EF

DE = EF

6. Grasping point E′, transpose the flap with point E′, meeting point C. Place a stitch at the asterisk along line EF where it joines line DE, to align the flap and close the secondary defect (Figure 60C). Place another suture aligning line D′E′ with line BC to completely close the flap. Close the remaining flap as usual.

7. Repeat this flap, beginning at point B instead of point D, until you thoroughly understand its mechanics.

Z-PLASTY

The Z-plasty obtains its name from the fact that the transposition of two interlocking triangular flaps shapes a Z. Understanding the Z-plasty can be a challenging exercise in geometry. However, two main changes occur with the placement of the Z-plasty: (1) a change in the length of the wound, and (2) a change in the direction of the central line of the Z-plasty. The Z-plasty drawn in Figure 61 shows a lengthening of the common diagonal (sometimes called the contracted diagonal), as one use of this flap is to lengthen a contracture. The common diagonal changes direction to become the transverse diagonal by transposing the arms of the Z-plasty.

Figure 61
Z-plasty

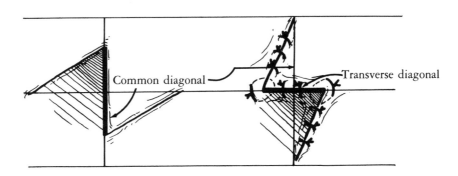

Two points in the construction of the Z-plasty are critical to its understanding and performance. These are angle size and length of the common diagonal (also referred to as the central member in some texts). Consider **angle size** first. As illustrated in Figure 62, the smaller the angles adjacent to the central member, the less the gain in length of the common diagonal. The greater the angles, the greater the gain in length. The angles adjacent to the central member for optimum performance of this flap should be 60 degrees. Figure 62 illustrates the effect of the changes in the size of the angles adjacent to the common diagonal of the Z-plasty, with the common diagonal length remaining constant. The percentage gains given are theoretical, and vary in actual practice. Studies have shown that the gain in length varies from 45 percent less to 25 percent more than the gain calculated geometrically, due to the biomechanical properties of the skin. The **length of the common diagonal** is also critical to the geometry of the Z-plasty. The greater the length of the central member, the greater will be the actual gain in length accomplished by the performance of the Z-plasty (Figure 63A). This lengthening occurs because, regardless of the angles, the arms of the Z-plasty must always be equal to the length of the common diagonal. The length of the common diagonal becomes important when considering the fact that to lengthen the common diagonal, the transverse diagonal (Figure 61) is consequently shortened. Tension is placed along the transverse diagonal in order to transpose the two triangles. If the common diagonal were too long, and the Z-plasty was placed in relatively inelastic skin, too much tension would be placed along the transverse diagonal. When this occurs (it is often done deliberately for cosmetic reasons) in addition to tension on the transverse diagonal, multiple Z-plasties can be used to achieve the same common diagonal lengthening with less of a shortening effect on the transverse diagonal. The effects are illustrated in Figure 63B.

Figure 62
Z-plasty: increase in common diagonal with change in angle

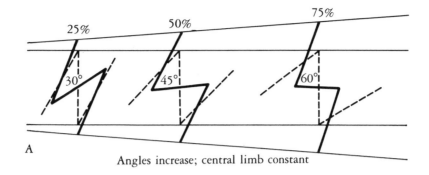

Angles increase; central limb constant

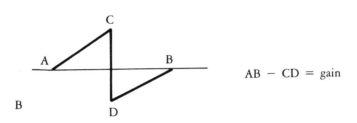

AB − CD = gain

Figure 63
Z-plasty: increase in common diagonal with increase in central member (angle remaining constant)

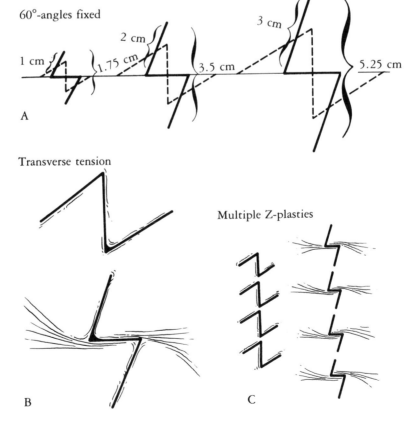

Figure 64 illustrates the actual performance of a 60-degree angle **Z**-plasty. The common diagonal of this **Z**-plasty is line BC, which is the line that will be lengthened. Line AD will be shortened. Remember that the arms of the **Z**-plasty adjacent to the 60-degree angles must be equal in length to the common diagonal. Therefore, AB must equal B'C', which equals C'D. Theoretically, this 60-degree angle **Z**-plasty will lengthen line BC by 50 percent. In performing the **Z**-plasty, it is important to pull in the direction of the open arrows shown in Figure 64B, as this will transpose or interchange the triangles. Pulling in the direction indicated also lengthens the common diagonal. It is important that the triangles be interchanged once the **Z**-plasty is cut and undermined. A common mistake is to place the triangles back in the position from which they originated. The triangles can also be moved by gingerly placing a skin hook in each tip (B and C in Figure 64) and forcing the transposition of the triangles.

EXERCISE 41: Z-PLASTY

1. Draw a 2 cm line on the pig's foot.
2. Refer to Figure 64 and draw limbs AB and CD as shown, using a caliper or a ruler. If a means of making a 60-degree angle accurately is not readily available, you can best estimate one by making a 90-degree angle and dividing it into thirds. Two of these will give you a fairly accurate estimate of a 60-degree angle.
3. After placing a dot at point B', cut the **Z**-plasty.
4. Undermine both arms of the **Z**-plasty completely.
5. Place a skin hook at the open arrows shown in Figure 64B, and pull. This should interchange the interlocking triangular flaps. You can make sure of the complete transposition of the flaps by making sure that the dot you placed at point B' has moved.
6. Place the key stitch in the center of the transverse diagonal, as illustrated in Figure 64.
7. Close the angles, using three-point corner (tip) stitches.
8. Finish the closure.
9. Use your ruler to measure the gain in length between points B and C shown in Figure 64. Theoretically, this gain in length should be about 50 percent.
10. Repeat this exercise, varying the angles and the length of line BC, until you feel comfortable with this method of tissue movement.
11. Repeat this exercise, but use multiple **Z**-plasties instead of one alone to lengthen the line, as shown in Figure 63C.

Figure 64
Performing a Z-plasty

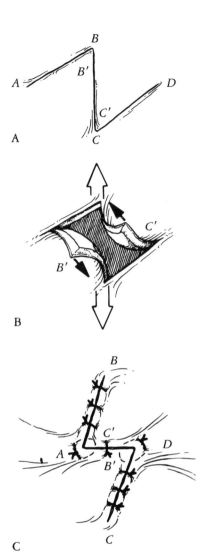

Practice Tests

TEST 1

1. Excise a circle of skin on the pig's foot.
2. Triangulate one end of the circle, and remove the triangle.
3. Create a **T**-type closure at the end of the circle opposite to that which you triangulated.
4. Undermine completely. Review the method for closing wounds of unequal length.
5. Use a different method to close each branch of the **T**.
6. Repeat this exercise until you feel comfortable with the procedure.

TEST 2

1. Excise a circular defect, as in Test 1.
2. Make this defect into a square.
3. Close this excision using a bilateral advancement flap (**H**-plasty). First draw and then excise the limbs of the **H**-plasty, elevate with a skin hook, and undermine (see Figures 43 and 44).
4. Place the key stitch to close the primary defect.
5. You have created wounds of unequal length. Close the upper left side following the rule of halves, the upper right side by removing a Burrow's triangle laterally, and the lower branches by removing a dog-ear or triangle centrally.
6. Finish the closure.

TEST 3

1. Excise a circular defect.
2. Design a rotation flap extending from one side of the circle.
3. Cut and undermine the arc of the rotation flap.
4. Place a stitch in the tip of the rotation flap, and move the flap so that the tension on the closures of the primary defect and secondary defect is shared.
5. Remove this stitch and place the key stitch to close the primary defect. You have now created a dog-ear and a wound with unequal sides.
6. Remove the dog-ear using an **M**-plasty.
7. Remove a triangle at the midportion of the longer side of the wound.
8. Finish the closure.

TEST 4

1. Excise a circular defect.
2. Close this excision using an **O-Z** double rotation flap. Diagram and cut the initial arcs of the **Z**.
3. Undermine and pull the tissue (see Figure 51). If there is too much

tension in the center of the wound, extend the sides of the rotation flaps.

4. Place the key stitch to close the primary defect. Wounds of unequal length result.
5. Close the left side by the rule of halves or by removing a lateral triangle.
6. Close the right side by removing a triangle from the center of it.
7. Finish the closure.

TEST 5

1. Excise a circular defect.
2. Close this excision using a bilobe double transposition flap. Design the bilobe flap, referring to Figure 55 if necessary.
3. Remember that the area under the initial lobe should be approximately two-thirds to three-fourths of the area of the circle. The area of the second lobe should be approximately one-half the area of the initial circle.
4. Cut along the lines you have diagrammed, elevate, and undermine.
5. Place the key stitch to close the secondary defect and align the flap.
6. Close the transposed flaps as desired, leaving a dog-ear at one edge of the circle initially cut as the primary defect.
7. Excise the dog-ear, using a hockey-stick dog-ear repair, triangulating the excess tissue, and widening the base of the flap.
8. Finish the closure.

TEST 6

1. Draw a circular defect on the pig's foot.
2. With a pen or gentian violet, make the circle into a parallelogram.
3. Go through the exercise of creating a Webster 30-degree angle flap by first extending one end of the parallelogram to create a 30-degree angle.
4. Draw the sides of the 30-degree angle by careful measurement.
5. Incise the drawn sides and undermine the flap. **Do not** make the **M**-plasty as in the classic example.
6. Close the secondary defect, aligning the flap.
7. Finish the closure.
8. Repeat the procedure for this flap until you are comfortable with its design and tissue movement.

TEST 7

1. Draw a circular defect on the pig's foot.
2. Imagine the circle as a very large square or parallelogram. From two

sides of the circle, directly opposite each other, design two rhombic flaps. The flaps should be equal in size on each side, as if they were a double rhombic flap.

3. Cut and undermine each side of the flap.

4. Close by placing two key stitches to close the two secondary defects.

5. The tissue should be transposed so that the two flaps meet in the center of the defect. Place a stitch joining the two flaps.

6. Finish the closure.

TEST 8

1. Draw a 3-cm line on the pig's foot. You will lengthen this line using Z-plasties.

2. Design three 60-degree angle Z-plasties (multiple Z-plasties) that will lengthen this line. Proceed with cutting and undermining the Z-plasties, as shown in Figures 63 and 64, but attempt to do this without referring back to those figures.

3. Transpose the tissue of the multiple Z-plasties, and anchor the flaps with a few stitches.

4. Remeasure the length of the initial line to prove that you have indeed lengthened it.

5. Repeat this exercise as many times as necessary to fully understand the principles behind the Z-plasty.

3 Advanced Techniques: Local Skin Grafts

Classification of Grafts

Free skin grafts refer to the moving of skin from one part of the body to another part of the body, severing the skin's local blood supply. Skin grafts are of two types: full-thickness skin grafts and split-thickness skin grafts (Figure 65). This chapter will explain the basics of skin grafting, first defining some terms used in skin grafting, and then discussing the full-thickness skin graft and the split-thickness skin graft.

The **full-thickness skin graft** refers to transfer of the epidermis and the complete dermis from their original site. After transplantation, the full-thickness skin graft more closely approximates normal recipient skin in color, texture, hair growth, and failure to contract than does the split-thickness skin graft. The full-thickness graft is usually smaller in area than the split-thickness graft, as the donor site is usually sutured for closure. The **split-thickness skin graft** refers to transfer of the epidermis and a portion of the dermis from the sight of origin. Depending on its depth, the split-thickness skin graft is divided into thin, medium, or thick layers (Figure 65). This division varies in thickness from 0.010 to 0.025 inch in the normal individual. The translucency of the graft and the bleeding pattern of the donor site also help to determine the thickness of the graft. As you might expect, the thin split-thickness graft will be more translucent than the thick split-thickness graft. With the thin split-thickness graft, the bleeding pattern at the donor site shows a high density of fine, small bleeding points. As a rule of thumb, the thicker the graft, the larger the bleeding points. The split-thickness skin graft, especially when on the thin side, will less closely resemble normal skin in color, texture, hair growth, and failure to contract than the full-thickness graft. Because most donor sites occur below the level of the clavicle, the color of split-thickness grafts is often yellowish white to tan. Hair growth, except in the case of a very thick split-thickness skin graft, does not occur. In general, the thinner the split-thickness skin graft, the more the graft will contract during its healing phase. Unlike the sutured donor site of a full-thickness skin graft, the donor sight of the split-thickness skin graft is left to reepithelialize. The **composite skin graft** refers to the transfer of full-thickness skin plus underlying tissue. The underlying tissue can be fat alone or can include cartilage as well. An example of a graft containing fat would be a plug used in hair transplantation. Composite skin grafts including cartilage are sometimes used for reconstructing the nasal ala.

Figure 65
Schematic of skin graft
thickness

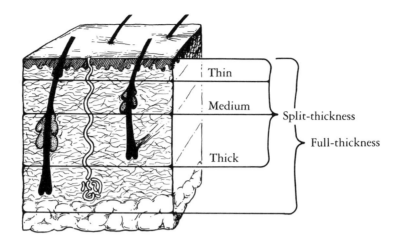

The **donor area** refers to the anatomic site from which graft skin is harvested. Donor sites vary depending on the type of skin graft to be performed, and will be discussed with each type individually. The **recipient site** is the bed of tissue on which the free skin graft is placed. The recipient bed must be vascular; in a qualitative sense, it should be vascular enough to produce granulation tissue spontaneously. Exposed bone, cartilage, tendon, and nerve are usually not good sites for graft survival, but the periosteum, perichondrium, peritenon, and perineurium all usually have sufficient blood supply to promote graft survival. Grafts can be helped to survive in small areas of avascular tissue by the process of bridging. The **bridging phenomenon** refers to graft survival from a small avascular area due to collateral vessel supply and ingrowth from the periphery of the graft and recipient bed. The bridging phenomenon is illustrated in Figure 66.

The recipient site, besides being vascular, must also be free of pathogens. Normal bacterial flora, especially in a noncompromised host, will not interfere with graft survival. However, even a small concentration of pathogens will usually cause free graft failure. The most common pathogens causing graft failure are coagulase-positive staphylococci and *Pseudomonas*. Beta-hemolytic *Streptococcus*, even in small amounts, will cause graft dissolution. Therefore, grafts must be harvested in a sterile fashion and placed on a vascular recipient bed that has been carefully cleansed of pathogens.

Contraction occurs in two fashions. The first is wound contraction, a normal function of wound healing, which refers to the decrease in circumference of the wound (recipient bed) as it heals. In general, the thinner the skin graft, the more wound contraction will occur; the thicker the skin graft, the less the wound contraction. Contraction of the graft also occurs. Full-thickness skin grafts contract less than split-thickness skin grafts. In general, the thicker the graft, the less graft contraction occurs. Contraction can begin to occur as early as ten days after the graft, and usually is not complete until six months later.

Graft take refers to the process that must occur for free skin grafts to survive. Graft take depends on the ability of the skin to have its blood supply severed and then reformed without direct reattachment. There are three major factors in the success of skin grafts. The first, previously discussed, is a vascular recipient bed free of pathogenic bacteria. The second is the vascularity of the graft itself. Thin split-thickness grafts

Figure 66
Bridging

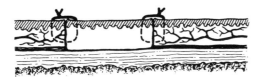

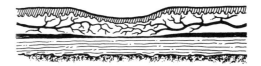

A   Graft placed on small avascular defect revascularized by ingrowth of
     peripheral vessels.

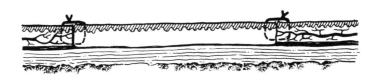

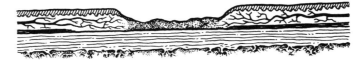

B   Graft placed on large avascular defect poorly revascularized.

are more vascular on their undersurface than thick split-thickness or thick full-thickness grafts. This difference in vascularity is because thin grafts have a very rich capillary network. Therefore, the survival of a split-thickness skin graft that is thin is higher than that of one which is thick, or than a full-thickness skin graft. The third factor affecting graft take is maintenance of contact between the skin graft and the recipient bed. A thin capillary network is formed almost immediately between a graft and its bed, which serves like a glue to hold the surfaces together. Problems that occur when proper contact is not maintained include improper tension on the graft, a collection of fluid (consisting of blood, serum, and purulent material) beneath the graft, and movement of the graft on its bed. Proper tension must be placed on the graft when suturing to maximize the contact between the graft and the recipient bed, yet not "strangle" the graft. Fluid must not be allowed to accumulate under the graft, and therefore meticulous hemostasis prior to placement of the graft is critical. If there is a serous ooze, the graft can be punctured, creating small fenestrations that allow for drainage. Immobilization of the graft can be accomplished using several methods which range from a tie-over type of dressing to basting stitches (these will be discussed with each grafting technique).

The vascularization of skin grafts is too broad a topic for detailed discussion here. However, two terms that are commonly used should be mentioned. **Plasmatic imbibition** refers to the initial fibrin "glue" that attaches the graft to the recipient bed. Nutrients to the graft are supplied from the plasma, probably by means of diffusion through the thin fibrin network. This creates a state somewhat like that of an in vivo tissue culture. Plasmatic imbibition occurs within the first twenty-four hours. The second common term is **inosculation of blood vessels,** referring to the growth of the vascular buds into and through the fibrin network, binding the skin to the recipient site. These vascular buds grow from the recipient bed and probably also from the grafted skin, and unite to form the early vascular network between the skin graft and its recipient bed. Inosculation of blood vessels usually begins around forty-eight hours after the graft is placed.

Full-Thickness Skin Grafts

By definition, the full-thickness skin graft is the free transfer of epidermis and complete dermis from one site to another. This is illustrated in Figure 65. Full-thickness skin grafts in cutaneous surgery are used principally on the head and neck region, but they can also be used on extremities to provide thicker coverage. Probably the most common site for a full-thickness skin graft is the nasal tip. In general, the benefits of the full-thickness skin graft are several. They provide coverage for a wound more quickly than healing by spontaneous granulation and with less surgical morbidity than often occurs with a flap. At times, defects exist that cannot be easily covered by a flap because of their location and size. Full-thickness skin grafts can provide the best cosmetic result in such cases. The nasal tip again is a good example.

Advantages of the full-thickness skin graft are mainly due to its thickness. Because it includes the full thickness of the dermis, this graft often provides the best color, texture, and thickness match. The full-thickness graft may also move hair-bearing skin because the dermal adnexal structures are intact. It also contracts less than does the split-thickness graft, and requires no special equipment for its performance. **Disadvantages** of full-thickness skin grafts are due to the special conditions necessary for graft survival. When full-thickness skin is being transferred, the recipient bed must be in optimal condition to ensure a full take of the graft. Meticulous suturing and wound approximation are critical to cosmesis. The size of the full thickness graft is restricted because of the limited location of donor sites and the fact that such sites must be closed primarily.

The **donor sites** for full-thickness skin grafts are illustrated in Figure 67 (shaded areas). In general, they are located above the level of the clavicle. The skin at these sites has been exposed to the sun during the patient's lifetime, and gives a better chance of color and texture match than does skin below the clavicle that has not been sun exposed. If the surgeon looks at donor sites considering the limitations and advantages of each, proper choice of donor skin can be made for the defect that must be closed. Characteristics of the recipient bed beside vascularity include location, depth of the defect, exposed avascular structures (e.g., bone, cartilage, or tendon), and skin color and texture. The donor site for the graft should be selected to best match these features.

Figure 67
Donor sites for full-thickness skin grafts

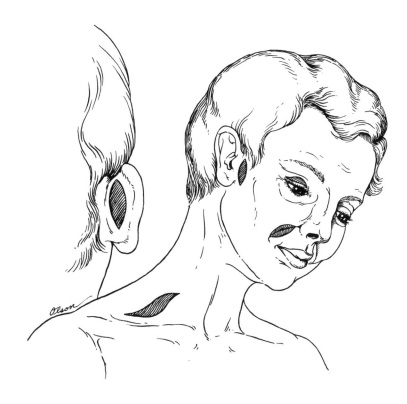

The eyelid as a donor site provides the thinnest full-thickness skin graft, and is used primarily for grafting skin to the opposite eyelid. It has an excellent color and texture match as well as excellent thickness for a thin defect on the eyelid. Postauricular skin comes close to the thickness of the eyelid, that is, it is very thin. Postauricular skin texture is smooth, and a color match with eyelid skin, especially in females, is often very good. Such a graft is limited by the size of the donor site. Preauricular skin provides a thicker graft with characteristics similar to those of the postauricular graft in texture and color. This graft is limited to the width of the skin at the donor site, between the tragus and the beginning of hair-bearing skin on the cheek. Preauricular skin is an excellent graft for thicker nasal tip defects on nonsebaceous noses. This is particularly true in females. If the patient is elderly and has a redundant nasal labial fold, this provides an excellent donor site for skin to be grafted on the nasal tip. This is especially true in males, where a good texture and thickness match can be obtained. Again, size of the donor site is a limitation. Supraclavicular skin often provides a fine donor site for grafting, especially in males, as the donor site can be sutured and will usually be hidden under a shirt. In females, particularly those who wear strapless clothing, the site must be chosen carefully. In males, particularly those with sebaceous skin and evidence of solar elastosis, the supraclavicular area provides an excellent texture and color match. It also is an area where a larger graft can be harvested than from other donor sites. In general, color and texture of a donor site are more important in males, because they often have more sebaceous skin than females and do not usually wear makeup to hide any small variations in color.

The techniques for harvesting and placing a full-thickness skin graft are illustrated in Figure 68. The patient is anesthetized with local anesthetic in the recipient site as well as in the selected donor site. As mentioned earlier, donor site selection will depend on the skin characteristics previously discussed, as well as on the location of the recipient bed. Epinephrine can be used with the local anesthesia, but our standard practice is to dilute the concentration to 1 : 300,000 to 1 : 400,000 units. The recipient bed is prepared by cleansing it thoroughly with Hibiclens (antimicrobial skin cleanser) and obtaining spot hemostasis or pressure hemostasis, as necessary. With the recipient bed well prepared in a sterile fashion, a template is made to exactly fit the recipient defect. Anything from paper from a suture packet, to gauze, to telfa can be used

Figure 68
Techniques for full-thickness skin grafts

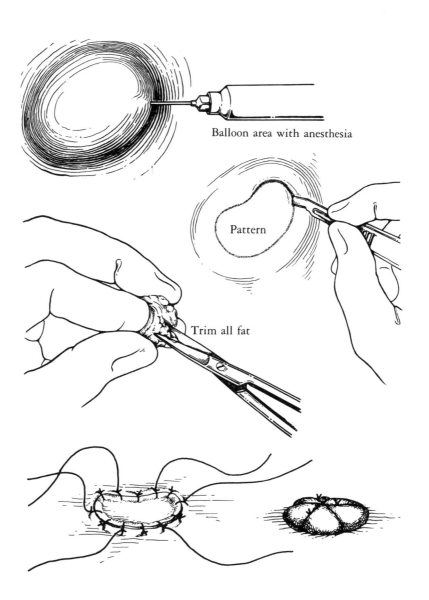

Balloon area with anesthesia

Pattern

Trim all fat

for the template. I prefer telfa, as it readily absorbs a small amount of serous ooze and is flexible enough to fit contours that will be grafted. The template is then cut and placed on the donor site. An outline can be drawn around the template, or an assistant can hold the template in place while a scalpel incision is made around it. The full thickness of skin is then removed. This can be done by attempting dissection at the level of the dermal-subcutaneous junction as the graft is removed, or by removing the graft and subcutaneous fat as you would in removing a lesion. I prefer the latter technique, as it is quicker, simpler, and a donor site must be excised to the level of fat in order to be closed anyway. The graft must then be kept moist; saline-impregnated gauze serves this purpose well. There is a critical period of time of approximately one-half hour at room temperature following graft removal during which the graft should be defatted and placed. The graft should be cooled if you anticipate a time lapse before joining the graft to the recipient bed. The donor site is then made into a geometric closure (usually an ellipse), is undermined, hemostasis is obtained, and the defect is closed with sutures. This is often done by an assistant while the graft is being defatted, or by the surgeon while the assistant defats the graft. The graft is best defatted by first placing the moist tissue epidermis side down on your finger and using sharp dissection scissors, removing all fat meticulously from the undersurface of the graft. When this has been done, you can place the graft on the recipient bed. If the template was accurate, the graft should fit exactly.

The graft is then sutured in place using one of a variety of techniques. My technique is to anchor the graft with six to eight interrupted nylon sutures, leaving one end of the suture long for a final tie-over dressing. I then place small interrupted stitches, using 6-0 Davis & Geck mild chromic or 6-0 Ethicon D6000 sutures. These are chromic gut sutures that usually dissolve in 4 to 6 days, so that they are gone by the time the dressing is removed at 5 to 10 days. Such suturing allows for good approximation of the graft edge to the edge of the recipient site, and also allows the anastamosis of vascular channels to begin without later disruption by suture removal. The edge of the graft can also be sutured to the recipient site using a running stitch. With the graft sutured in place, a bolus tie is placed over the dressing to anchor the graft to the recipient bed. This tie should be snug, not strangulating. I prefer to use Xeroform gauze directly over the sutured graft, with cotton or sponge placed on top of the Xeroform gauze. The sutures that were left long when suturing the graft are then tied over the Xeroform and cotton or sponge to produce the bolus tie-over dressing. A new material called N-Terface can be cut and placed between the graft and the Xeroform gauze to absolutely prevent sticking of the gauze to the graft at the time of removal. If the graft fits the recipient site well, a basting stitch can be used and a pressure dressing placed without the use of the tie-over dressing. Whatever method is used, it is important to obtain anchoring without motion of the graft over the recipient site to ensure the best conditions for graft take. The bolus tie-over dressing should be removed in approximately 1 week. At that time, the graft may be any color from pinkish, to pinkish-white, to black. Experience has shown that grafts that look the best at the time the tie-over dressing is removed can look black a week later, and end up surviving completely. A graft that is black at the time of dressing removal can also completely take. It is difficult to pass judgment on the final take of a graft until approximately one month after its placement.

The donor site is dressed using the usual sterile pressure dressing and following wound care instructions for a sutured wound. This means removing the pressure dressing in 24 to 36 hours, cleansing the suture line with hydrogen peroxide, and applying an ointment to keep the suture line moist. A telfa dressing is then placed. The sutures are removed in 5 to 10 days, depending on their location. Suture removal usually takes place at the same time the tie-over dressing is removed. Properly selected and sutured, the donor site usually heals with a fine, cosmetically indistinct scar.

As with any surgery, expectations of the patient and the surgeon must be carefully discussed beforehand. Grafts may fail, or may not take completely. They also will have a color and texture that usually does not exactly match surrounding skin. The patient must be counseled about these features of a skin graft before proceeding with the graft. It is also important to counsel the patient at the time the graft is placed concerning the appearance of the graft once the tie-over dressing is removed. If patients are told beforehand that a black graft can occur and can nevertheless result in a complete take, they are less likely to be upset at the time of dressing removal.

EXERCISE 42: FULL-THICKNESS SKIN GRAFTING

1. Draw a triangular or square defect on the pig's foot, and excise it.
2. Make a template using a piece of paper to exactly fit the geometric defect removed.
3. Place the template on the skin on another area of the pig's foot, and outline the graft to be removed.
4. Excise the graft.
5. Undermine and begin closing the primary defect. Once you are comfortable with the procedure for its closure, stop.
6. Place the removed graft with the epidermis down, on your finger, and remove any fatty tissue from the undersurface, using small dissecting scissors.
7. Place the graft on the hypothetical recipient site and anchor it with 4–6 interrupted nylon stitches, leaving one end long. Then anchor it with small interrupted stitches.
8. Place a hypothetical tie-over dressing, using whatever material you have available. When tying the dressing, use the long ends of the suture that are directly across from each other and snugly tie the loose ends of sutures, without strangulating. You have now performed a full-thickness skin graft.

Split-Thickness Skin Grafts

The split-thickness skin graft, by definition, is the free transfer of epidermis and a portion of dermis from one site to another (see Figure 65). Split-thickness grafts vary in thickness from 0.010 to 0.025 inch, and are classified as thin, medium, or thick, depending on the amount of dermis included with the graft. The characteristics of the split-thickness skin graft were discussed previously. These grafts can be used to cover a defect on any portion of the body.

The uses of the split-thickness skin graft are many. It can be a temporary coverage for wounds that are infected, are large, and would heal too slowly by spontaneous granulation, or in areas where a tumor with a chance of recurrence has been extirpated to observe the wound for a period of time prior to final reconstruction. Split-thickness grafts can cover large surgical defects, and can be used to line flaps that are used to cover full-thickness skin in the head and neck areas. The thin split-thickness graft, because of its increased vascularity, offers a better chance of take when placed in a relatively avascular bed (e.g., over periosteum or perichondrium).

The **advantages** of split-thickness skin grafts are several. They are technically easy to apply, as the edges need not be as carefully approximated as those of full-thickness skin grafts, and will often overlap. Large donor areas are available, allowing the coverage of large defects, especially with meshing of the graft. (Meshing will be explained later in this chapter.) They are successful, especially when thin, on almost any recipient bed and can be placed over compromised skin. **Disadvantages** of split-thickness skin grafts begin with their poor color and texture match. They usually heal with a whitish to yellowish tan color that rarely matches surrounding skin. The texture is usually smooth and there is little chance for survival of adnexal structures because full-thickness dermis is not included in the graft. Another disadvantage is that special equipment is often necessary, especially for large grafts. Lastly, the donor site is more difficult to care for, as it heals by secondary intention. This often takes more time than the sutured donor site of a full-thickness skin graft and can be quite painful.

The donor sites for split-thickness skin grafts are illustrated by the shaded areas in Figure 69. They are located where a broad area of tissue can be removed and hidden under clothing. The most common sites are the leg, usually the upper thigh, medial, posterior, and lateral. I prefer the anterior lateral of the thigh as a donor site for split-thickness grafting.

Figure 69
Donor sites for split-thickness skin grafts

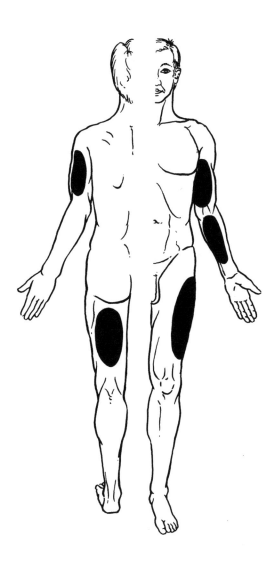

The arm can also be used, the most common areas being the lateral and medial upper arm and the flexural arm. The technique for the split-thickness skin graft is simple, although special instrumentation is often necessary; it is illustrated in Figure 70, using dermatomes. To begin, the recipient site must be again anesthetized, cleansed very well with an antiseptic such as Hibiclens, and meticulous hemostasis obtained. A split-thickness skin graft, especially when thin, can be placed on a relatively avascular bed. However, if possible, a bed can be left to granulate for a period of time prior to placement of the graft. This increases graft bed vascularity and decreases the depth of the defect to be closed. This is called a **delayed graft.** Instead of making a template, the size of the recipient bed is measured. After adding 20 to 25 percent to this measurement, outline this amount of skin to be removed on the donor site. The anterior-lateral thigh, because of its easy availability, is the most common donor site in my patients. This area is anesthetized with local anesthetic, cleansed well with Hibiclens, and rinsed with saline.

The instrumentation for performing split-thickness skin grafts varies. The simplest instruments used are scalpel blades or knives, such as the Weck blade, the Humby knife, or the Blair knife. If a small graft is necessary, a No. 10 Bard Parker blade can be used. There are two basic dermatomes, the electric dermatome and the drum dermatome. The Padgett-Hood dermatome is a drum dermatome preferred by some surgeons. It removes a piece of skin at a desired setting, depending upon pressure placed on the skin that wraps around the drum of the dermatome. I prefer the Brown electrical dermatome for harvesting skin. It is easy to use, the depth of the graft can be controlled by the caliper settings on the dermatome, and it can be autoclaved and reused. This instrument is illustrated in Figure 70.

Once the donor recipient beds have been anesthetized and cleansed, the dermatome is prepared. The undersurface of the dermatome as well as the area of the recipient bed are lubricated with sterile lubricating jelly or mineral oil. This allows easy and smooth passage of the dermatome over the skin. The dermatome setting is adjusted according to the desired thickness of the graft. Because the calibration of dermatomes is sometimes inaccurate, the setting can be approximately calibrated using the naked eye and bearing in mind that the back of a No. 15 Bard Parker blade is machined at approximately 0.015 inch. A set screw adjusts the width

**Figure 70
Dermatome—instrumen-
tation for split-thickness
skin grafts**

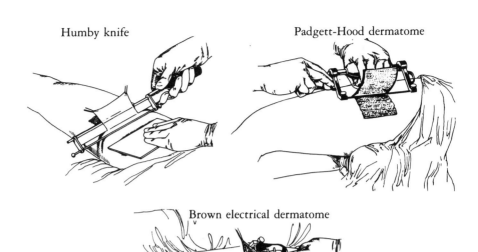

Humby knife

Padgett-Hood dermatome

Brown electrical dermatome

of the graft. The dermatome is placed on the skin, and with equal, moderate pressure, advanced approximately 1 cm. The assistant can then pick up the graft with hemostats as it begins to feed through the dermatome. The dermatome is advanced for the full measured length of the graft, and the graft is removed with a final upward motion of the dermatome.

The removed graft is then draped over the recipient bed and trimmed to fit approximately. It should be trimmed to be slightly larger than the recipient bed, due to subsequent contraction of the graft as explained earlier. Grafts tend to fold in on themselves, and care must be taken to have the cut underside in complete contact with the recipient bed. The graft is sutured and/or stapled in place, using interrupted or running sutures, and/or staples. Care must be taken to place the suture or staple at an angle, so that the graft is approximated along the full height of the wound edge. Often a graft is placed on a wound that is deeper than the thickness of the graft. In this case, the edge at the base of the wound must be carefully approximated, including the entire height of the defect (Figure 71). Staples are a very rapid way of obtaining such approximation in a split-thickness graft.

The graft is next anchored in place with several basting stitches, which are interrupted sutures placed through the graft and recipient bed to anchor and immobilize the graft. If the graft is placed over an area where anticipated fluid buildup will occur, the graft can be fenestrated with a No. 11 blade, or meshed (Figure 71). If the recipient site is large, the size of the graft can be increased by meshing. A sterile pressure dressing is then usually placed over the graft. If a graft is large, the patient may be instructed to roll the base of the graft with cotton-tipped applicators periodically, to prevent any fluid or air buildup between the graft itself and the recipient bed. The sutures and/or staples are usually removed after approximately 1 week. Split-thickness grafts, especially when thin, will often exhibit a better color and evidence of take more quickly than full-thickness grafts. The overlapping skin edge often becomes necrotic at approximately 10 to 14 days and can be trimmed. The donor site is relatively easy to care for. Immediately after the graft is removed, the assistant may place a telfa and cotton pressure dressing, anchored by an Ace bandage wrap. This dressing is left in place while the graft is anchored to the recipient site. Graft placement usually takes at least 30 minutes,

Figure 71
Technique for split-thickness skin grafts

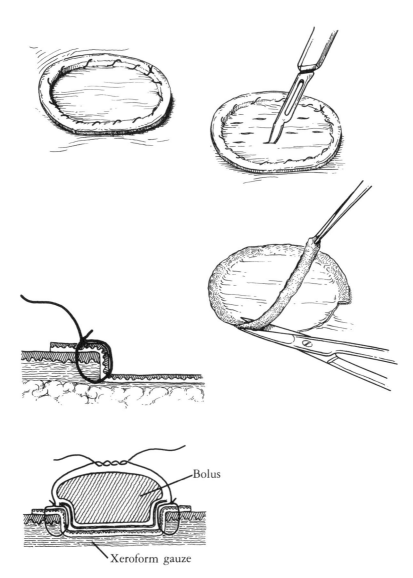

Bolus

Xeroform gauze

during which time the pressure from the Ace bandage wrap on the donor bed usually obtains hemostasis. If it does not, then aluminum chloride, or spot electrodessication as necessary, can be used. I prefer to use a membrane dressing (e.g., Op-Site) to cover the donor site area. This dressing is placed per the instructions for whichever dressing is used. The dressing should be approximately twice as large as the graft, as there is occasionally fluid buildup under this dressing. If buildup occurs, the dressing can be punctured with an 18-gauge needle, and the fluid withdrawn. A smaller piece of membrane dressing can be placed over the resulting puncture wound. If the patient is able to keep the large dressing in place, it will dramatically speed healing of the donor site, as well as alleviate discomfort at that site. If the dressing falls off, it can be reapplied, or the patient can begin routine dressing care, using moist occlusive dressing techniques.

The expectations for split-thickness skin grafts differ from those for full-thickness skin grafts. Split-thickness grafts are not as cosmetically elegant as full-thickness grafts. Their color-texture match is rarely excellent. These grafts often leave a depression in the area where they are placed, because they are usually thinner than the height of the defect they cover. However, they do provide good covering and more rapid healing than spontaneous granulation for most defects. Although split-thickness grafts, especially when thin, will exhibit contraction, they can limit the wound contraction that would occur in secondary intention healing. When used in cosmetically important areas, such as the head and neck, these grafts are often a temporary procedure to be followed by a more permanent, cosmetically elegant closure.

Appendixes

A. Anatomy

The whole of surgical anatomy is obviously beyond the scope of this book. However, the following diagrams stress important anatomic considerations in the planning of cutaneous surgery. The general anatomy and definitions of structures of the skin are critical (Figure 72). On the head and neck, the critical nerves and arteries of the face are illustrated; these include the facial nerve, supraorbital, infraorbital and mental nerves, and the arteries related to the external carotid system (Figure 73). Terminology of anatomic areas is also given. The anatomy of the hand and digit is illustrated in Figure 74. The musculature of the face is important, as it pertains to relaxed skin tension lines, and is illustrated.

Figure 72
Anatomy of the skin

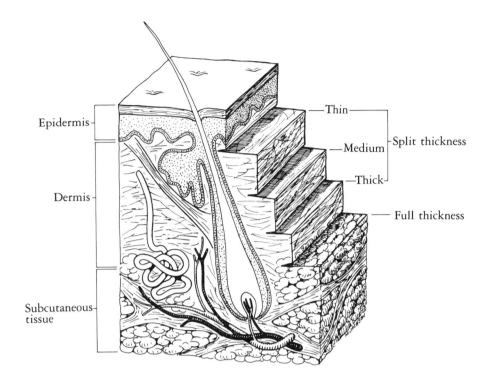

Figure 73
Anatomy of the face

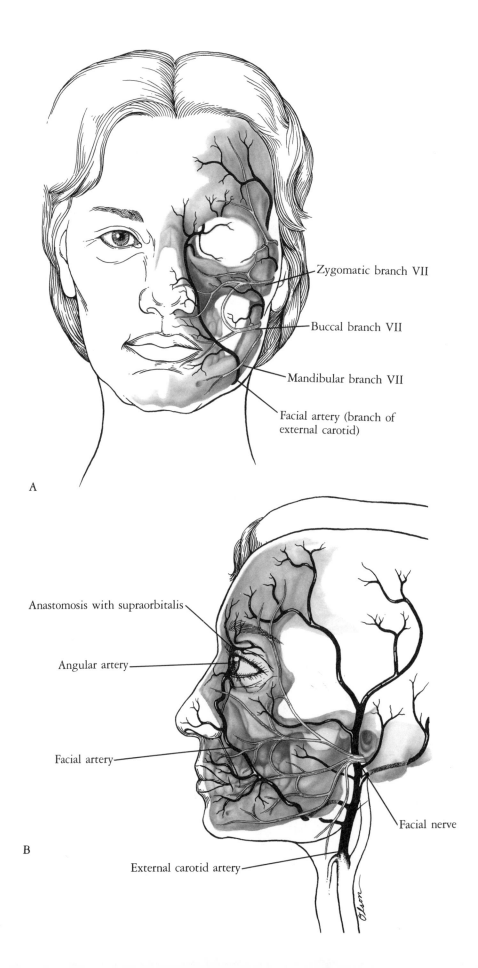

Zygomatic branch VII

Buccal branch VII

Mandibular branch VII

Facial artery (branch of
external carotid)

A

Anastomosis with supraorbitalis

Angular artery

Facial artery

Facial nerve

External carotid artery

B

Figure 74
Anatomy of the hand

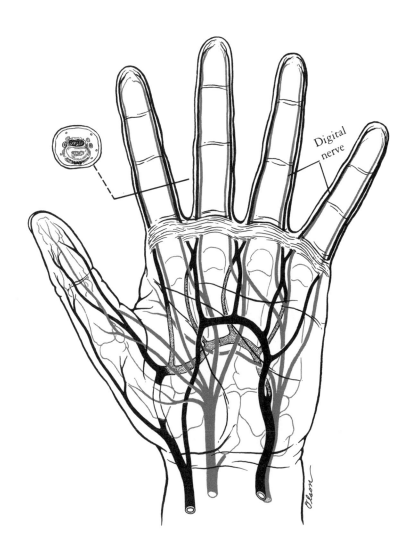

Digital
nerve

B. Relaxed Skin Tension Lines

Relaxed skin tension lines of the face and body are illustrated in Figures 75 and 76, respectively.

Figure 75
Relaxed skin tension lines: Face

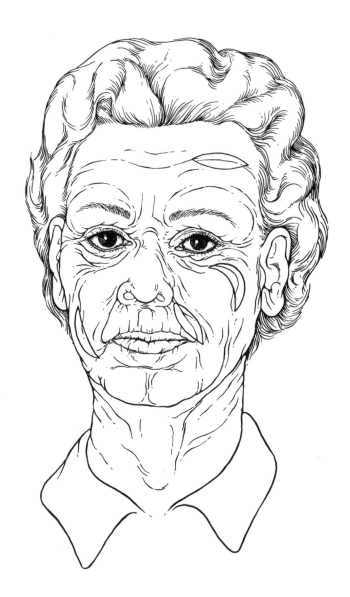

Figure 76
Relaxed skin tension
lines: Body

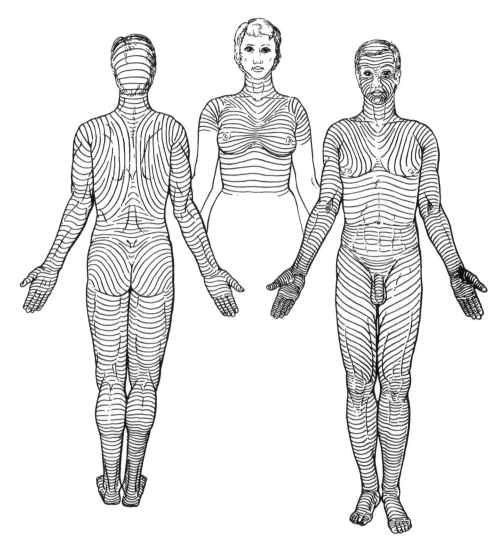

C. Local Anesthetics

For all of the cutaneous surgery described in this book, local anesthetics will suffice. A good understanding of their use is important before employing cutaneous surgical techniques on patients.

Cocaine was the first local anesthetic. Its use began around 1868. Cocaine was followed in the late 1800s by its derivative benzocaine. Benzocaine is still used topically as a 20% ointment. The first water-soluble ester anesthetic was procaine, whose use began around the turn of the century. The first amide anesthetic, called lidocaine (Xylocaine), was used in the early 1940s.

Before proceeding any further, some definitions are in order. **Regional anesthesia** refers to the temporary interruption of sensory nerve conductivity within a given area. Motor activity may or may not be involved, and the patient is conscious. **Local anesthesia** is the introduction of a nonvolatile substance at nerve endings to prevent the propagation of a nerve impulse. This can be done topically with surface application, or with local, direct infiltration of anesthetic into nerves in a limited area. A **field block** is the infiltration of anesthetic close to nerves around an operative field. A **nerve block** refers to direct injection of anesthetic into or along the course of a nerve at a distance from the operative site. The mechanism of action of the majority of local anesthetics is a block in the sodium (Na^+) flux, thus preventing a nerve fiber from reaching the threshold potential necessary to propagate a nerve impulse. In short, local anesthetics block depolarization. With the exception of the vasoconstrictor cocaine, all anesthetics are vasodilators. They also all enact vascular smooth muscle relaxation.

The properties of the ideal local anesthetic would be that of rapid onset of action with duration long enough to perform the procedure necessary. They would be of negligible systemic toxicity. The material would be stable and water soluble, and would be compatible with vasoconstrictors and body tissue fluids. Choice of local anesthetics, then, depends on the operation in question; the type of procedure, the site of the procedure, and the estimated duration of the procedure are all factors to consider. Which local anesthetic is used also depends on the patient's physical state, other illnesses, allergies, and the compatibility of the local anesthetic with any other medications the patient might be using.

The properties of the most common anesthetics are illustrated in Table 2. They fall into two general groups, esters and amides. The first group, esters, include cocaine, procaine, and pontocaine and are hydrolyzed in

Table 2. Local anesthetics for dermatologic surgery

Generic name	Trade name	Class	Onset of action	Average duration (min.)	Site of metabolism
Cocaine		Ester	Slow	120	Liver
Procaine	Neocaine, Novocain	Ester	Slow	50	Plasma
Pontocaine	Tetracaine, Pantocaine	Ester	Slow	175	Plasma
Lidocaine	Xylocaine, Seracaine	Amide	Rapid	100	Liver
Mepivacaine	Carbocaine	Amide	Intermediate	100	Liver
Bupivacaine	Marcaine	Amide	Intermediate	175	Liver
Etidocaine	Duranest	Amide	Rapid	200	Liver

plasma by pseudocholinesterase. This hydrolyzation produces PABA as a by-product, which cross-reacts with several other substances, including sulfonamides, thiazides, and sulfonylureas. The ester anesthesias are excreted by the kidney. The second group comprises amide compounds that include lidocaine, carbocaine, marcaine, and etidocaine. Amides are degraded in the liver by microsomal enzymes and are then excreted by it. The amide-linked anesthetics exhibit little cross-reactivity. Most local anesthetics, particularly lidocaine and carbocaine, contain preservatives. Parabens are the most common preservatives.

There are several techniques for administering local anesthesia. True local administration is the placement of anesthesia under a lesion to be removed. This was illustrated in Chapter 1 (see Figure 7). Often by raising a bleb of anesthesia, easy excision using scissors or scalpel can be performed. A field block refers to circumferential administration of anesthesia, that is, administration around a lesion. This often administers anesthetic to the central portion of the lesion not directly infiltrated, and is particularly useful in treating tumors where direct implantation of the needle through the tumor is undesirable, as in cutaneous squamous carcinoma. A nerve block is used in cutaneous surgery in some instances. The nerve block can be used on the face or digits. On the face, the most common nerves infiltrated for a nerve block are the supraorbital, infraorbital, and mental nerves, illustrated in Figure 77. These nerves are aligned along the midpupillary line. Nerve blocks are easy to perform with an understanding of the anatomy of the face, hand, and foot. The most difficult is the infraorbital nerve block. The infraorbital foramen has a bony hood, preventing direct access to the nerve. The nerve must therefore be approached from an inferior position, either by injecting through the skin, proceeding to the bone, and following up along the cheekbone under the hood, or from an intraoral approach. The same two approaches, percutaneous or intraoral, can be used for blocks to the mental nerve. The digital block, a common procedure in cutaneous surgery, is performed by injecting a small amount ($\leq$ 2 ml) of anesthesia around the base of the digit. Refer to Figure 74 in Appendix A for the location of the digital nerves. When injecting, you should begin on one side of the digit and slowly advance to the bone. Then inject circumferentially around that side of the digit. Repeat the procedure on the opposite side of the digit. Always withdraw as you go, to make sure that you are not injecting a vessel. When injecting the great toe, the same technique would be used. However, about a third of the time the area immediately under the nail bed will not receive anesthesia from a digital block, and must be locally infiltrated. For digital nerve blocks, no vasoconstrictor should be used.

Figure 77
Anesthesia: Nerve blocks on the face

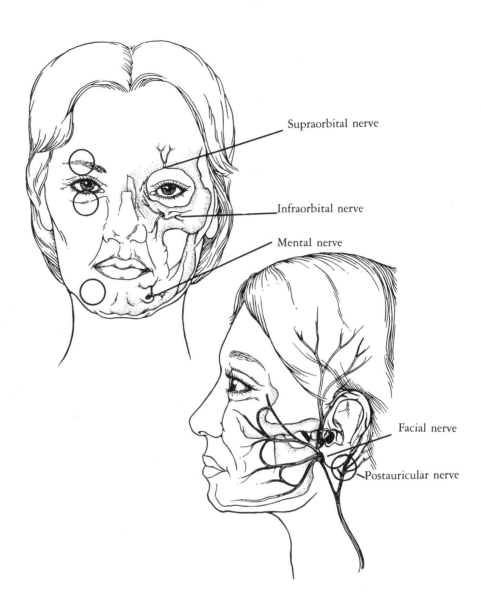

Supraorbital nerve

Infraorbital nerve

Mental nerve

Facial nerve

Postauricular nerve

Recommended dosages and dosage intervals follow certain rules, which depend on the maximum duration of action of the anesthetic. Dosage also depends on whether a vasoconstrictor, such as epinephrine, is used or not, as most vasoconstrictors prolong anesthetic action. For a 70 kg individual, the maximum amount of 1% lidocaine **with** epinephrine to inject every 2 hours approximates 50 ml. For the same individual the maximum dose of 1% lidocaine **without** epinephrine approximates 30 ml. In general, the total allowable dose for children is weight dependent and approximates one-third to one-half the adult dose.

Premedication for anesthesia is sometimes necessary, but I often find intravenous premedication to be unnecessary. Valium, given either orally or sublingually, is often sufficient. At times, intramuscular injections of analgesics such as meperidine (Demerol) or diazepam (Valium) are used. The following suggestions are helpful when using local anesthetics. The vasoconstrictor (e.g., epinephrine) can be mixed fresh. A stabilizer is added to the stock solution, which slightly acidifies it and causes stinging on injection. By mixing the vasoconstrictor fresh, you can adjust the dose of the vasoconstrictor necessary and thereby reduce pain on injection. Always inject through the smallest gauge needle possible. I rarely use a needle other than a 30 gauge. Warm the solution slightly in your hand before injection, and inject slowly. These steps all will lessen pain on injection.

There are some contraindications to local anesthetics. Severe blood pressure instability is one. A history of allergy to local anesthesia is another, although a true allergic reaction, especially to the amide anesthetics, is exceedingly rare. Most allergic reactions are of a vasovagal or syncopal nature. If the patient has a true, documented allergic reaction to local anesthetics, there are two substitutes I find useful. Antihistamines (e.g., diphenhydramine [Benadryl]) can be used. Dilute diphenhydramine to 12.5 mg/ml with normal saline, and inject. This causes vasodilatation, and if a vasoconstrictor is desired, add a small amount of epinephrine in the desired concentration. The affects of this anesthetic will last for approximately one half hour and will cause sedation. The injection of normal saline alone can also work as an anesthetic for a very short period of time. With both of these methods of anesthesia, onset of action is longer, there is increased pain with the injection, and duration of action is brief. Psychologic instability and liver or renal disease (affecting amides and esters

Table 3. Toxic reactions to local anesthetics

System	Toxic reaction
Central nervous system	Dizziness, drowsiness
	Tinnitus, difficulty focusing, slurred speech, muscle twitching, shivering
	Tonic seizure
	Depression with respiratory arrest
Cardiac/respiratory	Depression
Peripheral vascular	Vasodilatation

respectively) may also affect the dose of anesthesia used. The use of monamine oxidase (MAO) inhibitors and phenothiazines should be avoided with concomitant use of local anesthetics.

There are several general toxic effects with the use of local anesthetics (Table 3). Overdosage can cause generalized numbing, with tingling of the tongue usually the earliest sign. Accidental intravenous injection can occur. The most common generalized toxic effect is a vasovagal response to injection of the anesthetic. Systemic reactions are rare unless intravenous injection has occurred; these include central nervous system (CNS) effects, such as dizziness and drowsiness, tinnitus, slurred speech, muscle twitching, cardiorespiratory depression, and peripheral vascular vasodilatation. Local toxic effects include muscle necrosis, transient (motor) defects that often last longer than the sensory effect of the anesthesia, and bruising and edema at the injection site.

The concept of adding vasoconstrictors to local anesthetics is an important one. The most commonly used is epinephrine, in a concentration of 1 : 100,000 units. Studies have shown, however, that epinephrine can be diluted up to 1 : 600,000 units and still be effective. The vasoconstrictor decreases the absorption of the anesthesia, making more of the drug available locally. This action of the vasoconstrictor produces a more effective anesthetic using a smaller volume of drug, prolongs duration of anesthetic action, and decreases the systemic toxicity of the same dose of local anesthesia. Addition of vasoconstrictors also reduces bleeding and makes hemostasis easier. When using a vasoconstrictor, always wait 5 to 7 minutes before beginning surgery, as the initial effect of epinephrine is vasodilatation. Vasoconstrictors are indicated in highly vascular areas, when using a very concentrated anesthetic, and when using a local anesthetic of relatively high toxicity. In my practice, vasoconstrictors are used extensively. There are exceptions, including their use for peripheral nerve blocks, use on digits of the hand or foot, and use on the glans penis. On the tip of the nose, helix, globule of the ear, and other relatively avascular structures, I use epinephrine, but dilute the concentration. True contraindications to vasoconstrictors include labile hypertension and/or severe cardiovascular disease, peripheral vascular disease (especially in nerve block anesthesia), early pregnancy, and glaucoma. The other general contraindications for local anesthetics mentioned previously also apply.

Toxic effects of vasoconstrictors are usually excitatory. The most common side effect seen with the addition of vasoconstrictor to local anesthetics is a mild, transient tachycardia.

A thorough understanding of the topics discussed here, as well as of the properties of the local anesthetics that are given in Table 2, will help you in performing general cutaneous surgery. It is best to pick a local anesthetic that you will use consistently in your practice. The most commonly used local anesthetic is lidocaine (Xylocaine). It is an amide anesthetic with little cross-reactivity, and its average duration of action is appropriate for most procedures. Lidocaine is relatively inexpensive, and has a very rapid onset of action. In my practice I use mepivacaine (Carbocaine) for some nerve blocks (e.g., on the penis). I also use cocaine as a topical applied anesthetic in the nose, both for its anesthetic effect and its vasoconstrictor effect on nasal mucous membranes.

D. Wound Closure Materials: Sutures and Staples

Historically, many materials have been used to approximate wounds. As early as 5000–3000 BC, eyed needles were used to pass materials through wounds. By 2000 BC, bone needles were regularly used. Materials connected to these needles included flax, hemp, fascia, hair, linen strips, reeds and grasses, and other available exotic materials. Tying locks of scalp hair into knots to close scalp wounds was common during battles, and is still employed today as a temporary measure in some busy emergency rooms.

Natural products such as silk, cotton, linen, and catgut served as suture materials until the 1940s. During this decade, nylon and dacron became the first synthetic materials to be made into suture. Later, polyethylene, polypropylene, polyglycolic acid, and polyglycan 910 were developed and used in suture, adding to the surgeon's armamentarium.

Characteristics of the ideal suture material include superior tensile strength, good knot security, excellent handling characteristics, nonallergenic tissue reaction, resistance to infection, and eventual absorption when tissue repair has reached satisfactory levels. Unfortunately, there is still no ideal suture material. However, by becoming familiar with the different characteristics of modern suture materials, the best choice for any wound closure can be made.

PROPERTIES

Sutures are generally divided into two groups: absorbable and nonabsorbable. The general properties of each are listed in Tables 4 and 5. There are certain properties of suture materials that are important to consider when choosing a suture. **Knot security** refers to the ability of the suture to maintain knot strength without slipping. Knot security is inversely proportional to the memory of the suture material. **Memory** refers to the ability of the suture to maintain its shape. Sutures of high memory are less pliable, maintain their original shape, and can be more difficult to use. Monofilament sutures are examples of sutures with good memory. **Tensile strength** is a term used to describe both suture material and tissue, and refers to the strength per unit area of suture or tissue. **Breaking strength,** on the other hand, involves a measurement of strength per unit width of suture, and thus differs from tensile strength. Skin and fascia are examples of tissues of great tensile strength. Theoretically, suture materials need not have greater tensile strength than the wound being closed. **Tissue reactivity,** the ability of the suture to cause

Table 4. Properties of absorbable sutures

Suture type	Tensile strength	Wound security (days)	Tissue reaction	Knot security
Plain gut	+ +	5–7	+ + + +	+
Chromic gut	+ +	10–14	+ + +	+ +
Polyglycolic acid (Dexon)	+ + +	25	+ +	+ + +
Polyglycan 910 (Vicryl)	+ + +	30	+ +	+ + +
Polydioxanone (PDS)	+ + + +	60–90	+	+ + + +

Key: + = low; + + = moderate; + + + = high; + + + + = very high.

Table 5. Properties of nonabsorbable sutures

Suture type	Tensile strength	Wound security	Tissue reaction	Knot security
Silk	+	+	+ + + +	+ + + +
Dacron polyester (Mersilene)	+ +	+ + +	+ + +	+ + + +
Braided nylon (Nurolon)	+ +	+ +	+ + +	+ + +
Nylon	+ + +	+ + +	+ +	+ +
Polypropylene (Prolene)	+ + + +	+ + + +	+	+

Key: + = low; + + = moderate; + + + = high; + + + + = very high.

a local inflammatory response, can be critical. Maximum tissue reactivity occurs between the second and seventh day after suture implantation. Tissue reactivity occurs to some degree with all suture materials, although it is markedly less with monofilament sutures. Tissue reactivity for all sutures is given in Tables 4 and 5. **Wound security** refers to the strength of the wound over time. It is a reflection not only of wound healing but also of the tensile strength, knot security, and other characteristics of the suture material. With absorbable sutures, it is also a reflection of their loss of tensile strength over time. Wound security depends on both the original tensile strength of the suture and the rate of suture absorption.

ABSORBABLE SUTURES

Table 4 illustrates the absorbable sutures and their properties. **Plain gut** (catgut) is made from sheep intima and historically has been the longest available and best known suture. Plain gut maintains significant tensile strength for approximately 4 to 5 days. Wound security provided by this material is essentially gone in 14 days. Plain gut also causes the greatest amount of tissue reaction of the absorbable sutures.

Chromic gut is plain gut that has been treated by exposure to chromic salts in an attempt to retard its absorption into tissue. It has somewhat better wound security, with more delayed absorption, than plain gut. Its tensile strength is much less than that of the synthetic absorbable sutures. Like plain gut, chromic gut maintains wound security for approximately 14 days. There are two plain gut sutures on the market that deserve special attention because of their ability to be rapidly absorbed. One is manufactured by Davis & Geck and is called mild chromic gut; the other is manufactured by Ethicon and is a plain surgical gut known as D-6000. These are fast absorbing gut sutures and should be used on skin only. I often use them for suturing the edges of full-thickness skin grafts. **Polyglycolic acid** (Dexon) is one of the modern synthetic absorbable sutures. Polyglycolic acid is a high molecular linear copolymer of glycolic acid. It is a braided suture; it therefore lacks memory and is easier to handle than most monofilament sutures. However, because it is braided, it has a tendency to catch when pulled through subcutaneous tissue. It has a very high tensile strength, and maintains 50 percent of that tensile strength in tissue for up to 25 days. This suture material is generally totally absorbed in 90 to 100 days. It causes relatively low tissue reactivity, compared to plain gut. It is dissolved by enzymatic hydrolysis in the tissue, and does not involve phagocytosis.

Polyglycan 910 (Vicryl) is another synthetic polymer. It is the copolarization of a mixture of lactide and glycolide. It is available dyed (colored) and undyed, and is a braided suture. It is also available as coated Vicryl, where a Teflon-like coating has been added to the suture to help ease its passage through tissue. Like polyglycolic acid, polyglycan 910 possesses a very high tensile strength and maintains 50 percent of that tensile strength for approximately 30 days. It also requires 90 to 100 days for complete dissolution, and is removed by enzymatic hydrolysis without significant phagocytosis.

Polydioxanone (PDS) was the first monofilament absorbable suture. Manufactured by Ethicon, Polydioxanone has many of the properties of the monofilament sutures, including memory. However, it causes much less tissue reactivity than the braided sutures, passes more easily through skin, and maintains tensile strength for 60 to 90 days. When a buried absorbable suture, which must maintain tensile strength for the longest time (to permit collagen reorganization) is required, Polydioxanone is often the suture of choice.

NONABSORBABLE SUTURES

Table 5 gives the general properties of the nonabsorbable sutures. **Silk** has been a mainstay suture material for years. It has very little memory because it is braided, but therefore is very workable and ties secure knots. However, it does induce the most tissue reaction of any nonabsorbable suture. Silk has the lowest tensile strength of the nonabsorbable sutures. Its lack of memory and consequent good workability make it useful around the eyes, mouth, and orifices, and on the soles of the feet.

Dacron polyester (Mersilene) is a braided synthetic suture. It is a multifilament Dacron. It comes both dyed and undyed, making it useful in many areas. It causes less tissue reaction than silk, and can be used in the same anatomic areas as silk. **Nylon** was the first nonabsorbable monofilament suture. It has a good deal of memory, and therefore provides low knot security. It also has a good deal of tensile strength, providing very adequate wound security for skin. Its major asset is that it causes little tissue reaction, making it a valuable suture for routine use. **Braided nylon** (Nurolon) consists of fine nylon that is braided to give it tying characteristics closer to those of silk, while retaining the low reactivity of nylon. Its tensile strength is similar to nylon's. However, the knot security of braided nylon is poor and several knots are required to prevent slipping.

Monofilament sutures in general have several advantages over braided sutures. Synthetic monofilament sutures cause markedly less wound infection compared to braided sutures, as they are not colonized by bacteria; they can thus be used safely in contaminated wounds. This property, coupled with their high tensile strength and low tissue reactivity, make them an excellent cutaneous suture. Synthetic monofilament sutures are more difficult to use because of their high memory; however, with practice the surgeon can overcome this problem. Ethicon has recently released a new monofilament nylon suture, called "pliabilized" nylon. This material has been pretreated, and comes from the packet wet. Both these factors reduce the suture's memory, providing approximately the workability of a braided suture. The treatment process causes an approximately 15 percent loss of tensile strength, but this factor is usually not significant in cutaneous surgery. **Polypropylene** (Prolene) is a monofilament suture developed more recently than nylon. It consists of semisynthetic polypropylene polymer, and has extremely low tissue reactivity, even less than nylon. Polypropylene has slightly higher memory than monofilament nylon; however, polypropylene's workability may be improved with the future release by Ethicon of a pliabilized polypropylene. Polypropylene is manufactured as both a clear suture and a blue suture. The blue makes it easily visible, especially in hair-bearing skin, which is often gray, black, or blond. The clear version is useful as a permanent buried suture.

SURGICAL NEEDLES

Modern cutaneous surgery does not warrant the use of needles that require threading, produce large holes, and necessitate passing a double strand of suture through the wound. Modern suture material is swaged onto the needle to allow use of a smaller diameter needle as well as of a single strand of suture passing through tissue. Various types of needle tips are available. In almost all cutaneous surgery, a reverse cutting needle is preferred. This needle has a cutting edge on the outside of the curve, which actually makes a small cut in the tissue to allow smooth passage of the needle and suture. Since the cut is made away from the wound edge, the suture does not tear through tissue as sometimes happens with conventional cutting needles that have the cutting surface on the inside of the curve. Precision point needles combine the most highly honed steel with the sharpest point and are reported to maintain sharpness for a longer period of time than other needles.

Needle nomenclature has evolved in a manner that makes no sense. The surgeon must learn through experience which needle he prefers and the terminology of the needle manufacturer. In my experience, for the most part, needles manufactured by the Ethicon Corporation have superior sharpness and maintain their sharpness longer than other needles. Therefore, I will present the Ethicon nomenclature.

Ethicon makes two series of needles, the F series and the P series. The FS code denotes "for skin," and the PS code "plastic skin." The "P" in any Ethicon needle nomenclature denotes "plastic." FS and PS needles are ⅜ of a circle. P series needles are semicircular. PC needles are precision pointed, finely honed needles. F series needles are not as finely honed and do not maintain their sharpness as well as P series needles. They are approximately one-third the cost of the P needles. You can be cost-effective in practice by using a needle of appropriate sharpness according to the location to be sutured. The cost of a packet of suture material varies more with the needle choice than with the choice of suture material.

CHOICE OF SUTURE

Choice of suture used in surgical wounds depends on several factors. Knowledge of basic wound healing is critical. In the first two weeks,

Table 6. Suture choice and timing for removal

Location	Size	Removal (days)
Face	5-0–6-0	4–7
Neck, extremities, scalp	4-0–5-0	10
Trunk	3-0–4-0	10–14

epidermal wound healing occurs, with very little dermal wound healing. There is increasing collagen production in a wound up to approximately day 42, and then collagen realignment and remolding proceeds for approximately 6 months, with total wound remodeling occurring for up to 18 months. Wound cleanness (lack of infection) also plays a role. Monofilament sutures are better tolerated in contaminated wounds than are braided sutures. The anatomic location of the wound is also important in suture choice. For most cutaneous surgery on areas not surrounding orifices or eyelids, or on palms or soles, monofilament sutures are preferred. However, their high memory and resulting rigidity can be a nuisance around eyelids, orifices, and areas such as the palms or soles, where pressure is placed on the fine ends of stiff monofilament suture. Suture size is an important variable. The sizes of sutures used in cutaneous surgery range from 0 to 8-0; 8-0 suture is the finest. The size of a suture depends on the specific diameter necessary to produce a defined tensile strength. Therefore, the diameters of sutures of different materials for the same size category will vary. For example, a 5-0 silk suture will be greater in diameter than a 5-0 polypropylene suture, because the innate tensile strength of silk is lower. In general, the smaller sutures (5-0 and 6-0) are used cosmetically for areas on the face, where tissue is under less tension. The 3-0 and 4-0 sutures are used more commonly on the torso and the extremities. Very strong sutures are used in special circumstances, such as the approximation of the galea in a scalp reduction. Especially fine sutures (e.g., 7-0 and 8-0) are used for cosmetic procedures performed around the eyelids, such as a blepharoplasty.

Suture removal is another important consideration. Suture choice and timing of suture removal are presented in Table 6. Generally, the less time a suture is left in place to aid epidermal wound healing, the better the cosmetic result. Cosmetic result is also related to suture tightness and wound edge eversion. Tying the suture too tight can inhibit wound healing and leave undesired suture marks (railroad tracks) on the skin.

Table 7. Properties of three common brands of staples

Property	ETHICON (Proximate I, II)	3M (Precise)	U.S. Surgical (Premium)
Count	15, 35, 55	5, 10, 15, 30	12, 25, 35
Width (mm)			
Wide (width x height)	6.9 x 3.9	7.5 x 4.2	6.5 x 4.7
Regular (width x height)	5.7 x 3.9	5.0 x 3.5	4.8 x 3.4
Shape	box	heart	box
Arrow	yes	yes	yes
Precock	no*	yes	yes
Release	posterior	anterior	spring
Head	fixed*	fixed	rotates

*New unit will have precock and rotating head.

STAPLES

Staples are becoming increasingly useful for rapid, cosmetically acceptable cutaneous closure. Staples have always been known to give excellent wound closure because of the inert stainless steel used. Table 7 illustrates three of the most common staple manufacturers' products and several of the properties of stapling units. Other companies, such as Davis & Geck, and Decknitel, have entered the staple market, and there will be more entering it in the future.

As Table 7 reflects, staple units have several properties. Most have a fixed staple count per unit. This count varies as shown. Staples currently come in two sizes: regular-width and wide. The gauge of wire used varies somewhat, depending on the width of the staple. The shape of the staple is either a box, such as those made by Ethicon or U.S. Surgical, or heart-shaped, such as those made by the 3M Corporation. All staple units have an arrow that allows you to align the staple along the wound edges. The staple units with a precock, which shows the arms of the staple before stapling, allow for better and more accurate staple placement. The depth of staple penetration depends somewhat on pressure placed on the skin at the time of staple placement. The method of release of the staple from the unit varies. I prefer a spring release. Some units have to be slid anteriorly or posteriorly to release the staple from the staple gun, and this can be awkward. I also prefer a unit that has a rotating head, so that the position of the surgeon's arm does not have to change with the position of the head of the staple. This allows for easy staple placement in awkward situations and at close quarters. At the time of this writing, the U.S. Surgical Corporation unit best satisfies these requirements.

However, the Ethicon Corporation will have a stapler on the market soon that has similar features, but uses a smaller count staple. Other staple units with similar features should become available over a relatively short period of time.

Studies have shown that in comparisons for cosmesis, staples and sutures are equal. This is true for linear closures, grafts, and flaps. Staples, however, can be placed in literally seconds versus the several minutes required to place the same number of sutures. If staple manufacturing companies can keep the cost of staple units reasonable, these units may well begin to replace sutures in certain instances. Therefore, the cutaneous surgeon should become familiar with the use of staple units.

E. Hemostasis

Generalized bleeding is rarely an unmanageable problem in cutaneous surgery. A good history for bleeding dyscrasias and medication history for aspirin and aspirin-containing compounds will help prevent unwanted bleeding. The patient should stop taking aspirin and aspirin-containing compounds a minimum of 5 days prior to surgery. Inherited bleeding disorders are the only real contraindication to cutaneous surgery, as bleeding caused by warfarin (Coumadin) and/or aspirin derivatives can be controlled by anticoagulation, if the surgeon is prepared in advance. A platelet count above 50,000 is adequate for elective surgery. A **necessary** biopsy can be done as long as the platelet count is above 10,000.

Bleeding is either arterial or venous. The former is obvious and should be controlled as it occurs. Remember that if there is trouble with arterial bleeding, simple pressure at or proximal to the vessel will stop the bleeding temporarily while help is obtained. A larger vessel should be clamped with a hemostat and tied with a suture. This is true anywhere in cutaneous surgery, but especially on the lip. The tie can be done either by hand, off the tip of the hemostat, or with an instrument tie. The figure 8 stitch, illustrated in Figure 78, is a very nice way to obtain suture ligature. Minor arterial bleeding or venous bleeding can be controlled using the figure 8 stitch alone (without a hemostat) or electrosurgically. Using a bipolar electrosurgical unit with the patient grounded, a bleeding artery clamped with a hemostat or fine forceps can be coagulated by touching the instrument with current.

Most nonarterial bleeding in cutaneous surgery is controlled by electrical current or hemostatic solutions, which are listed below.

Figure 78
Hemostatic stitches: Figure 8 stitch

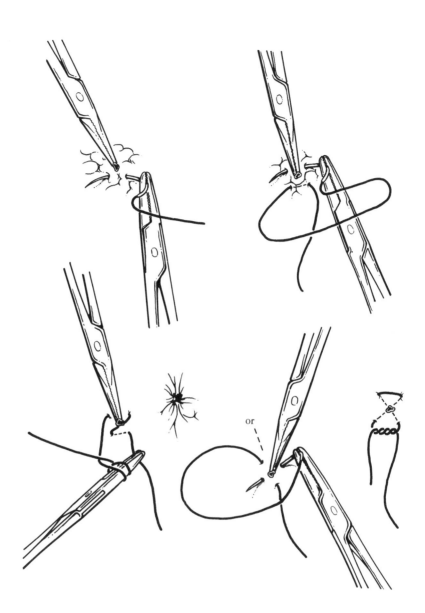

The **monopolar electrical unit** (Hyfrecator) is a low-amperage, high-voltage unit with active and dispersion electrodes in the same unit. Therefore, the patient does not have to be grounded. Monopolar units provide 90 percent of the electrosurgery needed in cutaneous surgery. They can be turned to lower settings for light electrodessication of vascular lesions, or to higher settings for electrofulguration for hemostasis. **Electrodessication** is tissue destruction by short, high-frequency sparks. This means actually touching the tissue with the electrode tip. **Electrofulguration** is tissue destruction by longer high-frequency sparks. This means *not* touching tissue with the electrode tip.

The **bipolar electrical unit** produces high-frequency current of higher amperage and lower voltage than the monopolar unit. It has one active and one dispersion electrode. The latter is usually a ground plate attached securely to the patient. This permits a marked concentration of current at the tip of the electrode, producing either electrocoagulation or cutting of tissue. **Electrocoagulation** is tissue destruction using bipolar current for hemostasis. **Electrocutting** is tissue destruction using bipolar current in a cutting mode.

Monsel's solution (ferric subsulfate) is a chemical cauterant used for good, fast hemostasis after most shave biopsies or excisions, or to control bleeding elsewhere. It is applied by a cotton-tipped applicator with pressure and rotation of the applicator tip. Because of the iron salt, it can cause tattooing. Therefore, it should not be used in cosmetically important areas.

Aluminum chloride solution acts similarly to but not as well as Monsel's solution. However, in concentrations approaching 40 percent it does not discolor the skin or produce tattooing as Monsel's solution can. Therefore, it is useful in cosmetically important areas.

Cellulose acetate (Oxycel or Gelfoam) is an absorbent cellulose material that aids hemostasis. It is useful for oozing not controlled by solutions, or after Mohs surgery. It is also useful in the mouth or on other mucosal surfaces.

Silver nitrate is available as silver nitrate sticks, which act as a chemical cauterant and are useful on mucosal surfaces and in the nose.

Index